PET/MRI: Clinical Applications

Editors

DREW A. TORIGIAN
ANDREAS KJÆR
HABIB ZAIDI
ABASS ALAVI

PET CLINICS

www.pet.theclinics.com

Consulting Editor
ABASS ALAVI

October 2016 • Volume 11 • Number 4

ELSEVIER

1600 John F. Kennedy Boulevard • Suite 1800 • Philadelphia, Pennsylvania, 19103-2899

http://www.pet.theclinics.com

PET CLINICS Volume 11, Number 4
October 2016 ISSN 1556-8598, ISBN-13: 978-0-323-46327-0

Editor: John Vassallo (j.vassallo@elsevier.com)
Developmental Editor: Meredith Clinton

PET Clinics (ISSN 1556-8598) is published quarterly by Elsevier Inc., 360 Park Avenue South, New York, NY 10010-1710. Months of issue are January, April, July, and October. Periodicals postage paid at New York, NY, and additional mailing offices. Subscription prices per year are $225.00 (US individuals), $366.00 (US institutions), $100.00 (US students), $255.00 (Canadian individuals), $412.00 (Canadian institutions), $140.00 (Canadian students), $260.00 (foreign individuals), $412.00 (foreign institutions), and $140.00 (foreign students). To receive student and resident rate, orders must be accompanied by name of affiliated institution, date of term, and the signature of program/residency coordinator on institution letterhead. Orders will be billed at individual rate until proof of status is received. Foreign air speed delivery is included in all Clinics subscription prices. All prices are subject to change without notice. POSTMASTER: Send address changes to PET Clinics, Elsevier Health Sciences Division, Subscription Customer Service, 3251 Riverport Lane, Maryland Heights, MO 63043. **Customer Service: 1-800-654-2452 (U.S. and Canada); 314-447-8871 (outside U.S. and Canada). Fax: 314-447-8029. E-mail: journalscustomerservice-usa@elsevier.com (for print support); journalsonlinesupport-usa@elsevier.com (for online support).**

Reprints. For copies of 100 or more of articles in this publication, please contact the Commercial Reprints Department, Elsevier Inc., 360 Park Avenue South, New York, NY 10010-1710. Tel.: 212-633-3874; Fax: 212-633-3820; E-mail: reprints@elsevier.com.

PET Clinics is covered in MEDLINE/PubMed (Index Medicus).

Contributors

CONSULTING EDITOR

ABASS ALAVI, MD, MD (Hon), PhD (Hon), DSc (Hon)
Professor, Division of Nuclear Medicine, Department of Radiology, Hospital of the University of Pennsylvania, University of Pennsylvania Perelman School of Medicine, Philadelphia, Pennsylvania

EDITORS

DREW A. TORIGIAN, MD, MA, FSAR
Clinical Director, Medical Image Processing Group; Associate Professor, Department of Radiology, Hospital of the University of Pennsylvania, Philadelphia, Pennsylvania

ANDREAS KJÆR, MD, PhD, DMSc
Professor, Department of Clinical Physiology, Nuclear Medicine & PET and Cluster for Molecular Imaging, Rigshospitalet and University of Copenhagen, Copenhagen, Denmark

HABIB ZAIDI, PhD, PD
Division of Nuclear Medicine & Molecular Imaging, Geneva University Hospital, Geneva, Switzerland

ABASS ALAVI, MD, MD (Hon), PhD (Hon), DSc (Hon)
Professor, Division of Nuclear Medicine, Department of Radiology, Hospital of the University of Pennsylvania, University of Pennsylvania Perelman School of Medicine, Philadelphia, Pennsylvania

AUTHORS

KIM FRANCIS ANDERSEN, MD
Department of Clinical Physiology, Nuclear Medicine & PET, Rigshospitalet, Copenhagen University Hospital, Copenhagen, Denmark

FARROKH DEHDASHTI, MD
Division of Nuclear Medicine, Edward Mallinckrodt Institute of Radiology; Alvin J. Siteman Cancer Center, Washington University School of Medicine, St Louis, Missouri

KATHRYN J. FOWLER, MD
Division of Abdominal Imaging, Edward Mallinckrodt Institute of Radiology; Alvin J. Siteman Cancer Center, Washington University School of Medicine, St Louis, Missouri

KENT P. FRIEDMAN, MD
Section Chief, Division of Nuclear Medicine, Department of Radiology, New York University Langone Medical Center, New York, New York

AMIT GUPTA, MD
Fellow in Radiology (Nuclear Medicine), Department of Radiology, University Hospitals Case Western Reserve University, Cleveland, Ohio

OTTO M. HENRIKSEN, MD, PhD
Chief Physician, Department of Clinical Physiology, Nuclear Medicine & PET, Rigshospitalet, Copenhagen, Denmark

KARL ERIK JENSEN, MD, DMSc
Department of Diagnostic Radiology, Rigshospitalet, Copenhagen University Hospital, Copenhagen, Denmark

ANDREAS KJÆR, MD, PhD, DMSc
Professor, Department of Clinical Physiology,
Nuclear Medicine & PET and Cluster for
Molecular Imaging, Rigshospitalet and
University of Copenhagen, Copenhagen,
Denmark

IAN LAW, MD, PhD, DMSc
Professor, Chief Physician, Department of
Clinical Physiology, Nuclear Medicine & PET,
Rigshospitalet, Copenhagen,
Denmark

ANNIKA LOFT, MD, PhD
Department of Clinical Physiology,
Nuclear Medicine & PET, Rigshospitalet,
Copenhagen University Hospital, Copenhagen,
Denmark

LISBETH MARNER, MD, PhD, DMSc
Staff Specialist, Department of Clinical
Physiology, Nuclear Medicine & PET,
Rigshospitalet, Copenhagen,
Denmark

STEPHAN G. NEKOLLA, PhD
Department of Nuclear Medicine, Technical
University Munich, München,
Germany

RAJ MOHAN PASPULATI, MD, FSAR
Professor of Radiology, Division of Abdominal
Imaging, Department of Radiology, University
Hospitals Case Western Reserve University,
Cleveland, Ohio

SUNE FOLKE PEDERSEN, PhD
Department of Clinical Physiology, Nuclear
Medicine & PET and Cluster for Molecular
Imaging, Rigshospitalet and University of
Copenhagen, Copenhagen, Denmark

IVAN PLATZEK, MD
Attending Physician, Department of Radiology,
Dresden University Hospital, Dresden,
Germany

MARIA ROSANA PONISIO, MD
Division of Nuclear Medicine, Edward
Mallinckrodt Institute of Radiology,
Washington University School of Medicine,
St Louis, Missouri

SAMUEL L. RICE, MD
Radiology Resident, Division of Nuclear
Medicine, Department of Radiology, New York
University Langone Medical Center, New York,
New York

RASMUS SEJERSTEN RIPA, MD, DMSc
Department of Clinical Physiology, Nuclear
Medicine & PET and Cluster for Molecular
Imaging, Rigshospitalet and University of
Copenhagen, Copenhagen, Denmark

CHRISTOPH RISCHPLER, MD
Department of Nuclear Medicine, Technical
University Munich, München, Germany

DREW A. TORIGIAN, MD, MA, FSAR
Clinical Director, Medical Image Processing
Group; Associate Professor, Department of
Radiology, Hospital of the University of
Pennsylvania, Philadelphia, Pennsylvania

Contents

18F-Fluorodeoxyglucose (FDG) PET/MR imaging is feasible for initial staging and therapy response assessment in lymphoma. Although FDG PET/MR imaging is equivalent to FDG PET/CT for initial staging of lymphoma, not enough data are available with regard to other indications yet. Diffusion-weighted MR imaging is a promising addition to FDG PET/MR imaging, but has not been evaluated systematically.

18F-Fluorodeoxyglucose (FDG) PET/MR imaging does not offer significant additional information in initial staging of squamous cell carcinoma of the head and neck when compared with standalone MR imaging. In patients with suspected tumor recurrence, FDG PET/MR imaging has higher sensitivity than MR imaging, although its accuracy is equivalent to the accuracy of FDG PET/CT.

Hybrid imaging systems have dramatically improved thoracic oncology patient care over the past 2 decades. PET-MR imaging systems have the potential to further improve imaging of thoracic neoplasms, resulting in diagnostic and therapeutic advantages compared with current MR imaging and PET-computed tomography systems. Increasing soft tissue contrast and lesion sensitivity, improved image registration, reduced radiation exposure, and improved patient convenience are immediate clinical advantages. Multiparametric quantitative imaging capabilities of PET-MR imaging have the potential to improve understanding of the molecular mechanisms of cancer and treatment effects, potentially guiding improvements in diagnosis and therapy.

PET/computed tomography (PET/CT) is an established hybrid imaging technique for staging and follow-up of gastrointestinal (GI) tract malignancies, especially for colorectal carcinoma. Dedicated hybrid PET/MR imaging scanners are currently available for clinical use. Although they will not replace regular use of PET/CT, they may have utility in selected cases of GI tract malignancies. The superior soft tissue contrast resolution and depiction of anatomy and the functional information obtained from diffusion-weighted imaging (DWI) provided by MR imaging in PET/MR imaging are advantages over CT of PET/CT for T staging and follow-up of rectal carcinoma and for better characterization of liver lesions. Functional information from

DWI and use of liver-specific MR imaging contrast agents are an added advantage in follow-up of liver metastases after systemic and locoregional treatment. New radio-tracers will improve the utility of PET/MR imaging in staging and follow-up of tumors, which may not be [18F]-2-fluoro-2-deoxy-D-glucose avid, such as hepatocellular carcinoma and neuroendocrine tumors. PET/MR imaging also has application in selected cases of cholangiocarcinoma, gallbladder cancer, and pancreatic carcinoma for initial staging and follow-up assessment.

This article summarizes recent advances in PET/MR imaging in gynecologic cancers and the emerging clinical value of PET/MR imaging in the management of the 3 most common gynecologic malignancies: cervical, endometrial, and ovarian cancers. PET/MR imaging offers superior soft tissue contrast, improved assessment of primary tumor involvement because of high-resolution multiplanar reformats, and functional MR techniques such as diffusion-weighted MR imaging and dynamic contrast-enhanced MR imaging. This article discusses the challenges, future directions, and technical advances of PET/MR imaging, and the emerging new multimodality, multiparametric imaging techniques for integrating morphologic, functional, and molecular imaging data.

The introduction of hybrid PET/MRI systems allows simultaneous multimodality image acquisition of high technical quality. This technique is well suited for the brain, and particularly in dementia and neuro-oncology. In routine use combinations of well-established MRI sequences and PET tracers provide the most optimal and clinically valuable protocols. For dementia the [18F]-fluorodeoxyglucose (FDG) has merit with a simultaneous four sequence MRI protocol of 20 min supported by supplementary statistical reading tools and quantitative measurements of the hippocampal volume. Clinical PET/MRI using [18F]-fluoro-ethyl-tyrosine (FET) also abide to the expectations of the adaptive and versatile diagnostic tool necessary in neuro-oncology covering both simple 20 min protocols for routine treatment surveillance and complicated 90 min brain and spinal cord protocols in pediatric neuro-oncology under general anesthesia. The clinical value of adding advanced MRI sequences in multiparametric imaging setting, however, is still undocumented.

There is emerging evidence suggesting that PET/MR imaging will have a role in many aspects of musculoskeletal imaging. The synergistic potential of hybrid PET/MR imaging in terms of acquiring anatomic, molecular, and functional data simultaneously seems advantageous in the diagnostic workup, treatment planning and monitoring, and follow-up of patients with musculoskeletal malignancies, and may also prove helpful in assessment of musculoskeletal infectious and inflammatory disorders. The application of more sophisticated MR imaging sequences and PET radiotracers other than FDG in the diagnostic workup and follow-up of patients with musculoskeletal disorders should be explored.

PET/MR Imaging in Heart Disease   465

Christoph Rischpler and Stephan G. Nekolla

Hybrid PET/MR imaging is a complex imaging modality that has raised high expectations not only for oncological and neurologic imaging applications, but also for cardiac imaging applications. Initially, physicians and physicists had to become accustomed to technical challenges including attenuation correction, gating, and more complex workflow and more elaborate image analysis as compared with PET/CT or standalone MR imaging. PET/MR imaging seems to be particularly valuable to assess inflammatory myocardial diseases (such as sarcoidosis), to cross-validate PET versus MR imaging data (eg, myocardial perfusion imaging), and to help validate novel biomarkers of various disease states (eg, postinfarction inflammation).

PET/MR Imaging in Vascular Disease: Atherosclerosis and Inflammation   479

Rasmus Sejersten Ripa, Sune Folke Pedersen, and Andreas Kjær

For imaging of atherosclerotic disease, lumenography using computed tomography, ultrasonography, or invasive angiography is still the backbone of evaluation. However, these methods are less effective to predict the likelihood of future thromboembolic events caused by vulnerability of plaques. PET and MR imaging have been used separately with success for plaque characterization. Where MR imaging has the ability to reveal plaque composition, PET has the ability to visualize plaque activity. Together this leads to a comprehensive evaluation of plaque vulnerability. In this review, the authors go through data and arguments that support increased use of PET/MR imaging in atherosclerotic imaging.

Clinical PET/MR Imaging in Oncology: Future Perspectives   489

Andreas Kjær and Drew A. Torigian

In 2011, the first fully integrated commercially available clinical PET/MR imaging systems became available, and the imaging community thought that these scanners would replace PET/CT systems. However, today a disappointing number of less than 100 scanners have been installed worldwide. The question, therefore, arises regarding what the future clinical applications of PET/MR imaging will be. In this article, the authors discuss ways in which PET/MR imaging may be used in future applications that justify the added cost, predominantly focusing on oncologic applications. The authors suggest that such areas include combined molecular and functional imaging, multimodality radiomics, and hyperPET.

PET CLINICS

PROGRAM OBJECTIVE

The goal of the *PET Clinics* is to keep practicing radiologists and radiology residents up to date with current clinical practice in positron emission tomography by providing timely articles reviewing the state of the art in patient care.

TARGET AUDIENCE

Practicing radiologists, radiology residents, and other health care professionals who provide patient care utilizing radiologic findings.

LEARNING OBJECTIVES

Upon completion of this activity, participants will be able to:
1. Review clinical applications of PET and MRI in lymphoma and other cancers.
2. Discuss the clinical use of PET/MRI in heart and vascular disease.
3. Recognize clinical applications for PET/MRI in musculoskeletal disorders.

ACCREDITATION

The Elsevier Office of Continuing Medical Education (EOCME) is accredited by the Accreditation Council for Continuing Medical Education (ACCME) to provide continuing medical education for physicians.

The EOCME designates this enduring material for a maximum of 15 *AMA PRA Category 1 Credit*(s)™. Physicians should claim only the credit commensurate with the extent of their participation in the activity.

All other health care professionals requesting continuing education credit for this enduring material will be issued a certificate of participation.

DISCLOSURE OF CONFLICTS OF INTEREST

The EOCME assesses conflict of interest with its instructors, faculty, planners, and other individuals who are in a position to control the content of CME activities. All relevant conflicts of interest that are identified are thoroughly vetted by EOCME for fair balance, scientific objectivity, and patient care recommendations. EOCME is committed to providing its learners with CME activities that promote improvements or quality in healthcare and not a specific proprietary business or a commercial interest.

The planning committee, staff, authors and editors listed below have identified no financial relationships or relationships to products or devices they or their spouse/life partner have with commercial interest related to the content of this CME activity:

Abass Alavi, MD, MD (Hon), PhD (Hon), DSc (Hon); Kim Francis Andersen, MD; Farrokh Dehdashti, MD; Anjali Fortna; Kathryn J. Fowler, MD; Kent P. Friedman, MD; Amit Gupta, MD; Otto M. Henriksen, MD, PhD; Karl Erik Jensen, MD, DMSc; Andreas Kjær, MD, PhD, DMSc; Ian Law, MD, PhD, DMSc; Annika Loft, MD, PhD; Lisbeth Marner, MD, PhD, DMSc; Stephan G. Nekolla, PhD; Raj Mohan Paspulati, MD, FSAR; Sune Folke Pedersen, PhD; Ivan Platzek, MD; Maria Rosana Ponisio, MD; Samuel L. Rice, MD; Rasmus Sejersten Ripa, MD, DMSc; Christoph Rischpler, MD; Erin Scheckenbach; Drew A. Torigian, MD, MA, FSAR; John Vassallo; Rajakumar Venkatesan.

UNAPPROVED/OFF-LABEL USE DISCLOSURE

The EOCME requires CME faculty to disclose to the participants:
1. When products or procedures being discussed are off-label, unlabelled, experimental, and/or investigational (not US Food and Drug Administration [FDA] approved); and
2. Any limitations on the information presented, such as data that are preliminary or that represent ongoing research, interim analyses, and/or unsupported opinions. Faculty may discuss information about pharmaceutical agents that is outside of FDA-approved labelling. This information is intended solely for CME and is not intended to promote off-label use of these medications. If you have any questions, contact the medical affairs department of the manufacturer for the most recent prescribing information.

TO ENROLL

To enroll in the PET Clinics Continuing Medical Education program, call customer service at 1-800-654-2452 or sign up online at http://www.theclinics.com/home/cme. The CME program is available to subscribers for an additional annual fee of USD $235.

METHOD OF PARTICIPATION

In order to claim credit, participants must complete the following:
1. Complete enrolment as indicated above.
2. Read the activity.
3. Complete the CME Test and Evaluation. Participants must achieve a score of 70% on the test. All CME Tests and Evaluations must be completed online.

CME INQUIRIES/SPECIAL NEEDS

For all CME inquiries or special needs, please contact elsevierCME@elsevier.com.

Preface
PET/MR Imaging: Clinical Applications

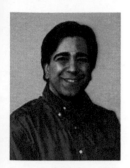
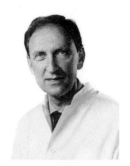
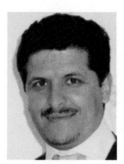
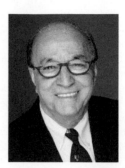

Drew A. Torigian, MD, MA, FSAR   Andreas Kjær, MD, PhD, DMSc   Habib Zaidi, PhD, PD   Abass Alavi, MD, MD (Hon), PhD (Hon), DSc (Hon)

Editors

Clinical PET/MRI systems have recently become commercially available, offering many advantages compared with PET/CT, leading to much enthusiasm in the medical community at large. Such advantages include a reduced exposure to ionizing radiation, superior soft tissue contrast resolution, and the capability to provide functional and multiparametric imaging data based on advanced MRI techniques (eg, diffusion-weighted imaging, dynamic perfusion imaging, magnetic resonance spectroscopy, or magnetic resonance elastography) that are complementary with the molecular data provided by PET. However, the higher costs, the slower scanning times with associated lower patient throughputs, the increased complexity, and the relative lack of diagnostic benefit of PET/MRI in some clinical applications relative to either PET/CT or independently acquired PET and MRI have somewhat dampened this initial excitement. Yet, it is likely that PET/MRI will still play an important future role in the clinical diagnostic imaging assessment of certain groups of patients with certain disease conditions, although such niche applications are still being defined. Additional technical challenges hampering quantitative imaging including the lack of consensus on reliable and accurate MRI-guided attenuation correction techniques are being addressed by active research groups in the scientific literature.

Therefore, in this issue of *PET Clinics*, we have enclosed a series of review articles that focus on clinical PET/MRI. In particular, clinical applications of PET/MRI for the evaluation of malignancy (including lymphoma, head and neck cancer, breast cancer, lung cancer, gastrointestinal tract cancers, and gynecologic cancers), brain disease, musculoskeletal disorders, and cardiovascular disease are discussed. We also briefly provide an article regarding our future perspectives on clinical PET/MRI in the oncologic setting. This issue nicely complements the April 2016 issue, "PET/MRI: Advances in Instrumentation and Quantitative Procedures," (Vol. 11, No. 2) edited by Dr Habib Zaidi.

We would like to thank all of the authors who contributed these articles, and we hope that the readers of these articles will learn much and apply what is learned to the future clinical practice of PET/MRI for the benefit of their patients.

Drew A. Torigian, MD, MA, FSAR
Department of Radiology
Hospital of the University of Pennsylvania
3400 Spruce Street
Philadelphia, PA 19104, USA

Andreas Kjær, MD, PhD, DMSc
Department of Clinical Physiology
Nuclear Medicine & PET
and Cluster for Molecular Imaging
Rigshospitalet and
University of Copenhagen
KF-4012, Blegdamsvej 9
2100 Copenhagen, Denmark

Habib Zaidi, PhD, PD
Division of Nuclear Medicine & Molecular Imaging
Geneva University Hospital
CH-1211 Geneva, Switzerland

PET Clin 11 (2016) xi–xii
http://dx.doi.org/10.1016/j.cpet.2016.07.001
1556-8598/16/© 2016 Published by Elsevier Inc.

Abass Alavi, MD, MD (Hon), PhD (Hon), DSc (Hon)
Department of Radiology
Hospital of the University of Pennsylvania
3400 Spruce Street
Philadelphia, PA 19104, USA

E-mail addresses:
Drew.Torigian@uphs.upenn.edu (D.A. Torigian)
akjaer@sund.ku.dk (A. Kjær)
habib.zaidi@hcuge.ch (H. Zaidi)
abass.alavi@uphs.upenn.edu (A. Alavi)

¹⁸F-Fluorodeoxyglucose PET/MR Imaging in Lymphoma

Ivan Platzek, MD

KEYWORDS

• PET/MR imaging • FDG • Lymphoma • Staging • Recurrence

KEY POINTS

- ¹⁸F-Fluorodeoxyglucose (FDG) PET/MR imaging is equivalent to FDG PET/CT for initial staging in lymphoma and has high sensitivity and specificity for nodal lymphoma involvement.
- Initial results suggest that FDG PET/MR imaging is also feasible for therapy response assessment in lymphoma; no comparison with other modalities is available for this indication.
- The role of diagnostic MR imaging, and especially of diffusion-weighted MR imaging as part of FDG PET/MR imaging in lymphoma, has yet to be determined.

INTRODUCTION

This article reviews the use of ¹⁸F-fluorodeoxyglucose (FDG) PET/MR imaging for lymphoma imaging. Lymphomas are among those malignancies with the highest incidence worldwide.[1,2] They are a diverse group of malignancies originating in lymphatic cells, associated with greatly varying prognosis. Although classifications of lymphoma have changed several times during the last decades, the basic differentiation between Hodgkin's lymphoma (HL) and non-HL (NHL) remains. The World Health Organization classification of lymphoma is the most current and also most widely accepted lymphoma classification.[3]

Some risk factors for lymphoma have already been identified, and include ionizing radiation, human immunodeficiency virus infection or Epstein–Barr virus infection.[4] However, the majority of lymphoma cases are idiopathic.

Lymphoma often involves multiple lymph nodes and rarely other organs such as the lung, liver, or brain. Extranodal involvement is more common in NHL than in HL. Lymphoma patients present with a variety of symptoms, which depend on disease location and extent. Common symptoms include painless swellings caused by enlarged lymph nodes, weight loss, fever, and night sweats.

The final diagnosis of lymphoma is based on histology, which may be combined with immunophenotyping and fluorescence in situ hybridization. Tissue needed for histologic examination is most often acquired through excisional biopsy, although percutaneous biopsy may be used for more deeply located lymph nodes or masses.

The choice of therapy is influenced by lymphoma type, which is also a very important prognostic factor. The spread of the disease, that is, the location and extent of lymphoma involvement, is a further crucial factor for the choice of therapy.

ROLE OF IMAGING

Although histology is indispensable for diagnosing lymphoma, reliable evaluation of lymphoma spread in vivo is only possible using imaging. In patients with newly diagnosed lymphoma, imaging findings in combination with some clinical symptoms are categorized currently according to a modification of the Ann Arbor classification called

The author has nothing to disclose.
Department of Radiology, Dresden University Hospital, Fetscherstr. 74, Dresden 01307, Germany
E-mail address: ivan.platzek@uniklinikum-dresden.de

PET Clin 11 (2016) 363–373
http://dx.doi.org/10.1016/j.cpet.2016.05.001
1556-8598/16/$ – see front matter © 2016 Elsevier Inc. All rights reserved.

the Lugano classification.[5,6] This classification applies to both HL and NHL. The revised staging system for primary nodal lymphomas is summarized in **Table 1**.

Note that tonsils, Waldeyer's ring, and spleen are considered nodal tissue. Bulky disease refers to a single nodal mass 10 cm or larger or greater than one-third of the transthoracic diameter for HL. A variety of sizes have been suggested for NHL with limited evidence suggesting a single nodal mass 6 cm or greater as best for follicular lymphoma and a single nodal mass 6 cm or larger to 10 cm for diffuse large B-cell lymphoma, although none of the proposed sizes have been validated in the current therapeutic era.[6]

Imaging is also particularly important for assessment of therapy response in lymphoma and helps to identify nonresponders, who may benefit from changing the therapy protocol. Furthermore, imaging is also used in patients with suspected lymphoma recurrence. Imaging can also be used to identify suitable biopsy sites or to perform image guided biopsy in patients with suspected lymphoma but without palpable enlarged lymph nodes.

Currently, the most widely used imaging modalities for evaluation of lymphoma are computed tomography (CT) and PET/CT. MR imaging is mostly supplementary to CT and PET/CT, except for lymphoma of the central nervous system.

COMPUTED TOMOGRAPHY

Owing to its widespread availability, fast acquisition times, and relatively low cost, CT remains the most widely used modality for lymphoma imaging. In CT, the assessment of nodal and extranodal involvement in lymphoma is based on morphologic findings. For example, according to

the criteria introduced by the International Working Group,[7] lymph nodes with a maximum transverse diameter larger than 10 mm are to be considered as positive for lymphoma involvement, except for lymph nodes with a recognizable fatty hilum and thin cortex. The use of such morphologic criteria results in a relatively low specificity. CT's reliance on morphologic features is an even more important disadvantage in therapy response assessment. In patients with bulky disease, that is, multiple coalescing lymphomatous lymph nodes, masses often do not disappear completely, but often persist even after successful therapy. Based on CT, it is not possible to differentiate between residual lymphoma tissue and scar tissue in such cases.

PET/COMPUTED TOMOGRAPHY

PET/CT combines the anatomic information of the CT scan with information about tissue metabolism provided by PET. This combination is advantageous for many oncologic applications, such that PET/CT has completely replaced standalone PET. Because the majority of lymphomas are characterized by high FDG uptake,[8] FDG is the PET radiotracer of choice for lymphoma imaging.

Although less widely available than CT, FDG PET/CT is often used for lymphoma imaging owing to its unique advantages. Indications for FDG PET/CT in lymphoma patients include initial staging, therapy response assessment, and posttherapy surveillance.

FDG PET/CT is superior to other modalities in initial staging of most lymphoma types. It has better sensitivity and specificity in initial lymphoma staging than contrast-enhanced CT[9,10] and leads to upstaging in a substantial number of cases.[11] Furthermore, combined FDG PET/CT has higher

---

Table 1
Lugano classification for primary nodal lymphomas

Stage	Involvement	Extranodal (E) Status
I	One node or a group of adjacent nodes	Single extranodal lesions without nodal involvement
II	Two or more nodal groups on the same side of the diaphragm	Stage I or II by nodal extent with limited contiguous extranodal involvement
II bulky	II as above with "bulky" disease	Not applicable
III	Nodes on both sides of the diaphragm; nodes above the diaphragm with spleen involvement	Not applicable
IV	Additional noncontiguous extralymphatic involvement	Not applicable

Adapted from Carbone PP, Kaplan HS, Musshoff K, et al. Report of the Committee on Hodgkin's disease staging classification. Cancer Res 1971;31(11):1860–1; and Cheson BD, Fisher RI, Barrington SF, et al. Recommendations for initial evaluation, staging, and response assessment of Hodgkin and non-Hodgkin lymphoma: the Lugano classification. J Clin Oncol 2014;32(27):3062.

accuracy than standalone FDG PET[12] in initial staging.

Similarly, Freudenberg and colleagues[13] have shown that FDG PET/CT has superior accuracy for residual disease after therapy in lymphoma patients when compared with CT. FDG PET/CT was also shown to be useful in patients with clinical suspicion of lymphoma recurrence.[14]

Accordingly, current consensus papers recommend the use of FDG PET/CT for both initial staging and therapy response assessment in FDG-avid lymphoma.[6,15] FDG-avid lymphomas include the majority of lymphomas, except for chronic lymphocytic leukemia/small lymphocytic lymphoma, lymphoplasmacytic lymphoma/Waldenstrom's macroglobulinemia, mycosis fungoides, and marginal zone NHL.

MR IMAGING

Owing to relatively long acquisition times and limitations of anatomic coverage feasible in a single examination, MR imaging has long been a second-line modality in lymphoma imaging, mostly used in addition to CT or PET/CT for clarification of suspected extranodal involvement. The only important exception to this rule has been primary cerebral lymphoma,[16,17] because MR imaging is the method of choice for imaging of cerebral masses owing to its superior soft tissue contrast and versatility.

Advances in technology in the last decade have helped MR imaging to overcome limited anatomic coverage, and with modern MR imaging systems whole-body MR imaging examinations can be performed in a reasonable timeframe. In this context, diffusion-weighted MR imaging (DWI) of lymphoma has been of particular interest, because this method allows for indirect assessment of tissue cellularity in addition to the depiction of morphology.[18] Although initial results have been promising,[19] DWI is currently not used routinely for lymphoma imaging.

- Currently, FDG PET/CT is the imaging method of choice in FDG-avid lymphomas.
- CT is widely used in lymphoma imaging, but its reliance on morphologic criteria is a disadvantage, especially with regard to therapy response assessment.
- Currently, MR imaging is mostly supplementary to PET/CT or CT for lymphoma imaging, except for lymphoma of the central nervous system.

RATIONALE OF PET/MR IMAGING IN LYMPHOMA

Although FDG PET/CT is a major improvement in lymphoma imaging over earlier standalone methods, PET/MR imaging has the potential to advance lymphoma diagnostics even further owing to its greater versatility. Besides anatomic information, MR imaging also offers possibilities to evaluate tissue structure and metabolism not offered by CT, such as DWI or MR spectroscopy. The superior soft tissue contrast of MR imaging can be helpful to evaluate extranodal lymphoma involvement.

PET/MR imaging also offers a further reduction of radiation exposure compared with current PET/CT scanners, because MR imaging does not use ionizing radiation. Although radiation exposure in CT has been reduced greatly in the last decade, the reduced radiation exposure in PET/MR imaging may be relevant in pediatric patients or in patients undergoing multiple rounds of imaging (primary staging, therapy response assessment, etc).

PET/MR IMAGING TECHNIQUE

Patient preparation before FDG PET/MR imaging is identical to patient preparation in FDG PET or FDG PET/CT. Patients scheduled for FDG PET/MR imaging are instructed to fast for at least 6 hours before radiotracer injection. Blood glucose level is routinely controlled before FDG injection. If the blood glucose level is higher than 150 mg/dL, the examination is usually rescheduled. At the author's institution, FDG is administered intravenously about 60 minutes before the start of the PET scan. Based on previous experience with PET and PET/CT, the intravenously administered activity is 4.5 MBq FDG/kg body weight.[20] After injection, the patients are instructed to remain seated or reclining and to avoid excessive motion.

PET/MR imaging examinations consist of a fast MR imaging scan used for PET attenuation correction (attenuation MR imaging), a PET scan, and usually diagnostic MR imaging. In most lymphoma patients, PET coverage between the skull vertex and the upper thigh is sufficient.

The role of diagnostic MR imaging in PET/MR imaging of lymphoma and the optimal choice of sequences for this application have not been sufficiently evaluated. Attenuation MR imaging, which is a T1-weighted gradient echo scan (with or without the DIXON fat suppression technique), is generally optimized for fast acquisition and may be insufficient for detection of normal-sized lymph nodes, especially in patients with low body fat percentage or in specific locations such as the neck or mediastinum. T2-weighted images can ensure better lymph node delineation while requiring relatively little additional acquisition time, especially with current simultaneous PET/MR imaging systems. However, T2-weighted images are not expected to improve lymph node characterization compared with CT.

In contrast, DWI is a very interesting potential addition to FDG PET in lymphoma imaging, as it helps to differentiate between tissues of high and low cellularity. Signal intensity on diffusion-weighted sequences relates to the diffusion (ie, Brownian motion) of water molecules that is influenced by tissue structure, including tissue cellularity.[21] Diffusion is restricted markedly in many malignant diseases, including lymphoma, owing to high cell density.[18] Takahara and colleagues[22] have demonstrated that whole-body DWI during free breathing is feasible with adequate image quality.[22] Since then, several studies have confirmed that DWI is a promising method for lymphoma imaging,[23,24] as mentioned. PET/MR imaging allows combination of the information from FDG PET and DWI and also comparison of the 2 methods.

The value of DWI as a part of FDG PET/MR imaging in lymphoma has yet to be clarified. However, initial results by Giraudo and colleagues[25] suggest that DWI is a useful addition to FDG PET/MR imaging in lymphoma. At the author's institution, FDG PET/MR imaging in lymphoma also routinely includes DWI for research purposes.

FDG PET/CT in lymphoma generally does not include contrast-enhanced CT, because it does not provide significant additional information. By analogy, it can be assumed that contrast injection is not necessary in FDG PET/CT of lymphoma, except for cases with suspected extranodal disease.

PET/MR imaging technique

- Patient preparation in FDG PET/MR imaging is identical to FDG PET/CT.

- With regard to nodal involvement, the combination of FDG PET and attenuation MR imaging is equivalent to PET/CT.

- Initial results suggest that DWI is a useful addition to FDG PET/MR imaging

- In cases with suspected extranodal involvement, T2-weighted or contrast-enhanced MR images can be useful.

- Diagnostic brain MR imaging is indispensable in cases of suspected cerebral involvement.

IMAGE QUALITY AND RADIOTRACER UPTAKE QUANTIFICATION

With regard to PET image quality, currently available PET/MR imaging systems are generally equal to PET/CT. Available studies on PET/MR imaging in lymphoma have unanimously reported adequate PET image quality.[25,26] In addition, no negative effects of the PET hardware on MR image quality has been noticed.

Quantification of FDG uptake based on PET/MR imaging is also possible, but the results are scanner-dependent and not entirely comparable to uptake quantification based on FDG PET/CT. Interpretation of available data is complicated by the fact that in studies comparing PET/CT and PET/MR imaging, the time interval between radiotracer injection and PET data acquisition is not identical for both hybrid modalities. In a study comparing FDG PET/MR imaging and PET/CT in lymphoma, Giraudo and colleagues[25] found that maximum standardized uptake value (SUV_{max}) of suspected lymphoma lesions were significantly lower for PET/MR imaging compared with PET/CT, but are strongly correlated. In this case, the outcome is partly influenced by the fact that all PET/CT scans were performed after the PET/MR imaging (on the same day, after a single FDG injection).

Our relatively limited knowledge on radiotracer uptake quantification in PET/MR imaging is currently of little consequence, because the evaluation of PET images in lymphoma patients is based mainly on visual assessment.[15,27]

IMAGING FINDINGS

PET/MR imaging findings in lymphoma are a combination of features already known from the respective standalone imaging modalities.

Nodal involvement in lymphoma is characterized by enlarged lymph nodes with a round shape, which often lack of a fatty hilum. Such lymph nodes mostly display a strongly restricted diffusion and a homogenous gadolinium enhancement. In contrast with other malignancies, necrotic foci are uncommonly seen in nodal lymphoma. Multiple lymphomatous lymph nodes can form large, mostly homogenous, lobulated masses. The signal intensity of lymphomatous lymph nodes is typically higher than that of the signal intensity of the spinal cord on high b-value DWI[23] owing to restricted diffusion. However, there is significant overlap with benign lymph nodes in regard to signal intensity.

Extranodal lymphoma manifestations are often hypointense to the parenchyma of the affected organ on nonenhanced T1-weighted images and slightly hyperintense on T2-weighted images. They also mostly display homogenous gadolinium enhancement. Similar to nodal lymphoma, extranodal lymphoma lesions mostly show restricted diffusion. In organs that typically have high signal intensity on DWI, including liver, spleen, salivary glands, and testes,[28] focal lymphoma manifestations often have higher signal intensity than the surrounding parenchyma. Diffuse hepatic or splenic lymphoma involvement can cause hepatomegaly and splenomegaly, respectively. Osseous lymphoma is mostly osteolytic on CT, but can be limited to the bone marrow.

As mentioned, most lymphomas display high FDG uptake, both in affected lymph nodes and extranodal sites. The FDG uptake of lymphoma is typically higher in comparison with the surrounding structures.[20,29] Typical FDG PET/MR imaging findings in lymphoma are shown in **Fig. 1**.

Response assessment in lymphoma using FDG PET/MR imaging is currently mostly based on the so called "Deauville criteria," originally developed for FDG PET/CT.[15] The Deauville criteria are summarized in **Table 2**. According to these criteria, scores of 1 or 2 are compatible with complete metabolic response. A score of 3 is equivocal, but in most cases a sign of complete metabolic response. Scores of 4 or 5 with reduced, grossly unchanged, or increased FDG uptake relative to

baseline findings are compatible with partial metabolic response, no metabolic response, or progressive metabolic disease, respectively. A score of 5 also occurs when new lesions are present. The role of DWI in response assessment in lymphoma is currently the subject of research investigation and is not currently used in clinical decision making.

Typical PET/MR imaging findings in lymphoma

- Enlarged, homogenous lymph nodes.
- Lymph nodes or focal lesions with high FDG uptake.
- Multiple coalescing lymph nodes (bulky disease).
- Lymph nodes or focal lesions with restricted diffusion.

DIFFERENTIAL DIAGNOSIS IN PET/MR IMAGING OF LYMPHOMA

The differential diagnosis in lymphoma includes both malignant and benign disease conditions. Beside lymphoma, most other malignancies also have increased FDG uptake. In most cases, the primary tumor can be identified using FDG PET/MR imaging. Furthermore, the number and

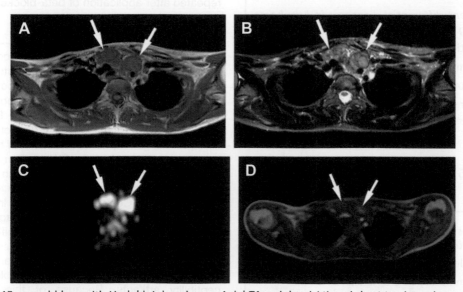

Fig. 1. A 15-year-old boy with Hodgkin's lymphoma. Axial T1-weighted (*A*) and short tau inversion recovery (*B*) nonenhanced images demonstrate marked lymph node enlargement in upper mediastinum (*arrows*). The high signal intensity of lymph nodes on axial high b-value diffusion-weighted imaging (*C*) indicates restricted diffusion. A corresponding combined ^{18}F-fluorodeoxyglucose (FDG) PET/MR image (*D*) shows high FDG uptake in lymphomatous lymph nodes.

Table 2
Deauville criteria

Score	FDG Uptake
1	No uptake
2	Slight uptake less than or equal to mediastinum
3	Uptake greater than mediastinum but less than or equal to liver
4	Uptake moderately higher than liver
5	Uptake markedly higher than liver and/or new lesions

distribution of enlarged lymph nodes can help to differentiate lymphoma from other malignancies. However, carcinoma of unknown primary can be mistaken for lymphoma if the primary tumor is not visible. In such cases, the final diagnosis is established based on histopathologic analysis.

Benign conditions that can cause lymph node enlargement and mimic lymphoma include infection, inflammation, and granulomatous diseases such as sarcoidosis.[30] Hyperplasia of the thymus can also have increased FDG uptake and be mistaken for mediastinal lymphoma.[31]

Important differential diagnoses in lymphoma imaging

- Infectious lymph nodes.
- Inflammatory lymph nodes.
- Granulomatous diseases.
- Carcinoma of unknown primary.

PITFALLS IN PET/MR IMAGING IN LYMPHOMA

The most relevant pitfalls in FDG PET/MR imaging include:

- Muscle FDG uptake,
- Inflammatory FDG uptake,
- Excreted FDG in ureters,
- Brown fat, and
- Metal artifacts.

Increased FDG uptake in benign processes may be misinterpreted as malignant lesions. In addition, MR imaging is prone to susceptibility artifacts that can, for example, be caused by metal implants and may obscure both anatomic structures and malignant findings. The most relevant pitfalls in FDG PET/MR imaging are summarized below.

Muscle Uptake

Resting muscles have a low FDG uptake, which can increase greatly with repeated muscle contraction. Even with careful patient preparation, increased FDG uptake is sometimes seen in muscles and can lead to false-positive findings. Careful comparison with MR imaging and multiplanar reconstruction of PET data helps to differentiate between intramuscular and extramuscular radiotracer uptake.

Brown Fat

In adults, brown fat is found mostly in the lower neck and upper mediastinum. It can show increased FDG uptake, especially in patients with low body fat percentage and in cold weather. The increased FDG uptake of brown fat is mostly symmetric, and coregistration with MR imaging in most cases allows one to differentiate this benign finding from lymphomatous lesions (**Fig. 2**). In cases with extensive FDG uptake in the brown fat, FDG PET/MR imaging can be repeated after application of beta-blockers.

Metal Artifacts

Metal implants or metallic foreign bodies can cause extensive susceptibility artifacts, which appear as areas of signal void accompanied by image distortion. Unfortunately, echoplanar sequences, which are routinely used in DWI, are especially prone to susceptibility artifacts. In patients with larger implants, evaluation of the areas surrounding the implants on DWI is often nondiagnostic. In such cases, turbo spin echo images, which suffer less from susceptibility artifacts, may be added. Comparison with PET images is even more important, because PET image quality is generally much less influenced by metallic objects when compared with MR imaging.

Gradient echo sequences, which are used for attenuation correction, are also vulnerable to susceptibility artifacts. Because of this, manual correction of attenuation maps may be needed in patients with metal implants. In cases with small susceptibility artifacts, automatic correction provided by the PET/MR imaging system is sufficient.

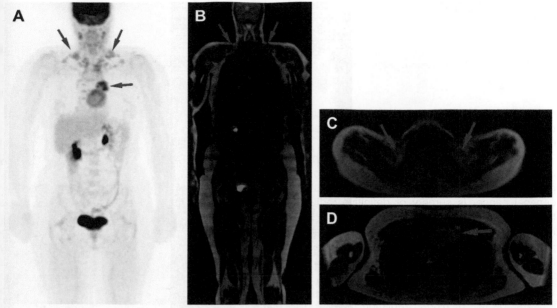

Fig. 2. A 48-year-old woman with follicular lymphoma. A lymphomatous mass (*red arrows*) in the anterior medi-astinum is seen on coronal maximum intensity projection (MIP) PET image (*A*) and combined axial ^{18}F-fluoro-deoxyglucose (FDG) PET/MR image (*D*). Also note increased symmetric FDG uptake within supraclavicular brown fat (*blue arrows*) on coronal MIP image (*A*) and on coronal (*B*) and axial (*C*) combined FDG PET/MR images.

INITIAL STAGING

FDG PET/MR imaging has been successfully established as an alternative modality in initial staging of lymphoma. For example, Platzek and colleagues[32] have shown that FDG PET/MR imaging has high sensitivity and specificity for nodal involvement in lymphoma. Although this study did not include comparison with other modalities, the results are very similar to previous results for FDG PET/CT.[33,34]

Furthermore, Heacock and colleagues[35] were able to show near complete agreement between FDG PET/MR imaging and FDG PET/CT with regard to lymph node involvement. In anal-ogous fashion, Giraudo and colleagues[25] found high levels of agreement between FDG PET/CT and PET/MR imaging for initial staging of lym-phoma. These results imply that FDG PET/MR imaging is equivalent to FDG PET/CT for initial lymphoma staging, at least with regard to nodal involvement. A typical patient who underwent FDG PET/MR imaging for initial staging of lym-phoma and follow-up examination is shown in **Fig. 3**.

Because extranodal involvement is less com-mon, it has not yet been evaluated systematically with PET/MR imaging. This is an area that may benefit from the superior soft tissue contrast of MR imaging.

TREATMENT RESPONSE ASSESSMENT

In an early pilot study, Platzek and colleagues[26] demonstrated that FDG PET/MR imaging is feasible for therapy response assessment in lym-phoma. However, a more detailed evaluation, including a comparison to PET/CT, is still lacking. Based on previous experience in initial staging, it can be expected that the information from PET images, which is currently essential for therapy response assessment in lymphoma, does not differ much between FDG PET/MR imaging and FDG PET/CT. The added value of DWI in PET/MR imaging for therapy response assessment has yet to be clarified (**Fig. 4**). Initial studies on standalone DWI imply a low specificity for residual disease.[36]

RECURRENT DISEASE

FDG PET/MR imaging has not been evaluated separately in patients with suspected lymphoma recurrence. Again, with analogy to initial staging, we do not expect major differences between FDG PET/MR imaging and FDG PET/CT in this clinical scenario.

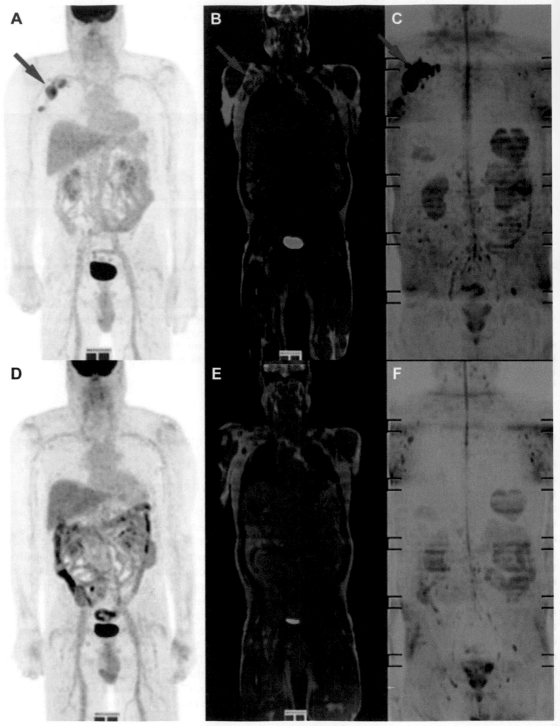

Fig. 3. A 62-year-old man with Hodgkin's lymphoma before and after 2 cycles of chemotherapy. Coronal MIP PET image (*A*), coronal combined ¹⁸F-fluorodeoxyglucose (FDG) PET/MR image (*B*), and inverted coronal maximum intensity projection (MIP) diffusion-weighted imaging (DWI) (*C*) show nodal lymphoma involvement in right axilla (*arrows*) with increased FDG uptake and restricted diffusion. After chemotherapy, Coronal MIP PET image (*D*), coronal combined FDG PET/MR image (*E*), and inverted coronal MIP DWI (*F*) show complete tumor response.

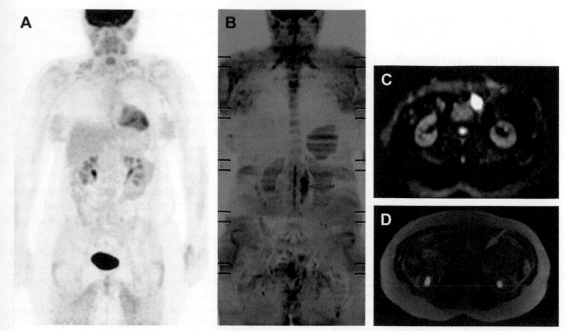

Fig. 4. A 52-year-old woman with diffuse large B-cell lymphoma who received 2 cycles of chemotherapy. Note discrepancy between coronal ^{18}F-fluorodeoxyglucose (FDG) PET maximum intensity projection (MIP) image (*A*), which shows no residual disease, and inverted coronal MIP diffusion-weighted image (DWI) (*B*), which shows left retroperitoneal lesion with restricted diffusion (*arrow*). Residual lymphoma (*arrow*) is also visible on the axial DWI (*C*), while axial fused FDG PET/MR image (*D*) shows that residual tissue (*arrow*) has very low FDG uptake.

RADIOTRACERS OTHER THAN ^{18}F-FLUORODEOXYGLUCOSE

Although FDG has long been the radiotracer of choice in lymphoma PET, alternative radiotracers have also been tested in lymphoma patients. The most important such example is ^{18}F-fluorothymidine, a radiotracer that shows strong uptake in actively proliferating tissues.[37] PET/CT with ^{18}F-fluorothymidine has shown promising results with regard to prognostic value.[38,39] To our knowledge, no reports of PET/MR imaging in lymphoma with radiotracers other than FDG have been published until now. Although all radiotracers evaluated using PET/CT can be used in PET/MR imaging, it should be noted that non-FDG PET radiotracers in lymphoma are still experimental.

SUMMARY

FDG PET/MR imaging is equivalent to FDG PET/CT in diagnostic performance for the initial staging of lymphoma, but with lower radiation exposure. Initial results suggest that DWI is a useful addition to FDG PET/MR imaging in initial staging of lymphoma. FDG PET/MR imaging is also feasible for therapy response assessment in lymphoma, but has not been compared with other modalities for this purpose.

What the referring physician needs to know:

- FDG PET/MR imaging is a new promising alternative to FDG PET/CT in lymphoma imaging, with lower radiation exposure.

- FDG PET/MR imaging is equivalent to FDG PET/CT in initial staging of lymphoma, at least with regard to nodal involvement.

- Initial results with FDG PET/MR imaging for therapy response assessment in lymphoma are promising, but the role of this new modality for this indication has yet to be validated.

REFERENCES

1. Jemal A, Bray F, Center MM, et al. Global cancer statistics. CA Cancer J Clin 2011;61(2):69–90.
2. Sant M, Allemani C, Tereanu C, et al. Incidence of hematologic malignancies in Europe by morphologic subtype: results of the HAEMACARE project. Blood 2010;116(19):3724–34.
3. Swerdlow SH, International Agency for Research on Cancer, World Health Organization. WHO classification of tumours of haematopoietic and lymphoid tissues. 4th edition. Lyon (France): International Agency for Research on Cancer; 2008. p. 439.

4. Grywalska E, Rolinski J. Epstein-Barr virus–associated lymphomas. Semin Oncol 2015;42(2):291–303.

5. Carbone PP, Kaplan HS, Musshoff K, et al. Report of the Committee on Hodgkin's Disease Staging Classification. Cancer Res 1971;31(11):1860–1.

6. Cheson BD, Fisher RI, Barrington SF, et al. Recommendations for initial evaluation, staging, and response assessment of Hodgkin and non-Hodgkin lymphoma: the Lugano classification. J Clin Oncol 2014;32(27):3059–68.

7. Cheson BD, Horning SJ, Coiffier B, et al. Report of an international workshop to standardize response criteria for non-Hodgkin's lymphomas. NCI Sponsored International Working Group. J Clin Oncol 1999;17(4):1244.

8. Weiler-Sagie M, Bushelev O, Epelbaum R, et al. (18) F-FDG avidity in lymphoma readdressed: a study of 766 patients. J Nucl Med 2010;51(1):25–30.

9. Schaefer NG, Hany TF, Taverna C, et al. Non-Hodgkin lymphoma and Hodgkin disease: coregistered FDG PET and CT at staging and restaging–do we need contrast-enhanced CT? Radiology 2004;232(3):823–9.

10. Pelosi E, Pregno P, Penna D, et al. Role of whole-body [18F] fluorodeoxyglucose positron emission tomography/computed tomography (FDG-PET/CT) and conventional techniques in the staging of patients with Hodgkin and aggressive non Hodgkin lymphoma. Radiol Med 2008;113(4):578–90.

11. Raanani P, Shasha Y, Perry C, et al. Is CT scan still necessary for staging in Hodgkin and non-Hodgkin lymphoma patients in the PET/CT era? Ann Oncol 2006;17(1):117–22.

12. Allen-Auerbach M, Quon A, Weber WA, et al. Comparison between 2-deoxy-2-[18F]fluoro-D-glucose positron emission tomography and positron emission tomography/computed tomography hardware fusion for staging of patients with lymphoma. Mol Imaging Biol 2004;6(6):411–6.

13. Freudenberg LS, Antoch G, Schutt P, et al. FDG-PET/CT in re-staging of patients with lymphoma. Eur J Nucl Med Mol Imaging 2004;31(3):325–9.

14. Taghipour M, Marcus C, Nunna P, et al. Follow-up FDG PET/CT in patients with non-Hodgkin lymphoma: value to clinical assessment and patient management. Clin Nucl Med 2016;41(2):e93–7.

15. Barrington SF, Mikhaeel NG, Kostakoglu L, et al. Role of imaging in the staging and response assessment of lymphoma: consensus of the International Conference on Malignant Lymphomas Imaging Working Group. J Clin Oncol 2014;32(27):3048–58.

16. Partovi S, Karimi S, Lyo JK, et al. Multimodality imaging of primary CNS lymphoma in immunocompetent patients. Br J Radiol 2014;87(1036):20130684.

17. Kickingereder P, Wiestler B, Sahm F, et al. Primary central nervous system lymphoma and atypical glioblastoma: multiparametric differentiation by using diffusion-, perfusion-, and susceptibility-weighted MR imaging. Radiology 2014;272(3):843–50.

18. Koh DM, Collins DJ. Diffusion-weighted MRI in the body: applications and challenges in oncology. AJR Am J Roentgenol 2007;188(6):1622–35.

19. Gu J, Chan T, Zhang J, et al. Whole-body diffusion-weighted imaging: the added value to whole-body MRI at initial diagnosis of lymphoma. AJR Am J Roentgenol 2011;197(3):W384–91.

20. Boellaard R, O'Doherty MJ, Weber WA, et al. FDG PET and PET/CT: EANM procedure guidelines for tumour PET imaging: version 1.0. Eur J Nucl Med Mol Imaging 2010;37(1):181–200.

21. Padhani AR, Koh DM, Collins DJ. Whole-body diffusion-weighted MR imaging in cancer: current status and research directions. Radiology 2011;261(3):700–18.

22. Takahara T, Imai Y, Yamashita T, et al. Diffusion weighted whole body imaging with background body signal suppression (DWIBS): technical improvement using free breathing, STIR and high resolution 3D display. Radiat Med 2004;22(4):275–82.

23. Kwee TC, van Ufford HM, Beek FJ, et al. Whole-body MRI, including diffusion-weighted imaging, for the initial staging of malignant lymphoma: comparison to computed tomography. Invest Radiol 2009;44(10):683–90.

24. Lin C, Luciani A, Itti E, et al. Whole-body diffusion-weighted magnetic resonance imaging with apparent diffusion coefficient mapping for staging patients with diffuse large B-cell lymphoma. Eur Radiol 2010;20(8):2027–38.

25. Giraudo C, Raderer M, Karanikas G, et al. 18F-Fluorodeoxyglucose positron emission tomography/magnetic resonance in lymphoma: comparison with 18F-fluorodeoxyglucose positron emission tomography/computed tomography and with the addition of magnetic resonance diffusion-weighted imaging. Invest Radiol 2016;51(3):163–9.

26. Platzek I, Beuthien-Baumann B, Langner J, et al. PET/MR for therapy response evaluation in malignant lymphoma: initial experience. MAGMA 2013;26(1):49–55.

27. Juweid ME, Stroobants S, Hoekstra OS, et al. Use of positron emission tomography for response assessment of lymphoma: consensus of the Imaging Subcommittee of International Harmonization Project in Lymphoma. J Clin Oncol 2007;25(5):571–8.

28. Kwee TC, Takahara T, Ochiai R, et al. Diffusion-weighted whole-body imaging with background body signal suppression (DWIBS): features and potential applications in oncology. Eur Radiol 2008;18(9):1937–52.

29. Shankar LK, Hoffman JM, Bacharach S, et al. Consensus recommendations for the use of 18F-FDG PET as an indicator of therapeutic response in patients in National Cancer Institute Trials. J Nucl Med 2006;47(6):1059–66.

30. Hollister D Jr, Lee MS, Eisen RN, et al. Variable problems in lymphomas: CASE 2. Sarcoidosis mimicking progressive lymphoma. J Clin Oncol 2005;23(31): 8113–6.

31. Sugawara Y, Fisher SJ, Zasadny KR, et al. Preclinical and clinical studies of bone marrow uptake of fluorine-1-fluorodeoxyglucose with or without granulocyte colony-stimulating factor during chemotherapy. J Clin Oncol 1998;16(1):173–80.

32. Platzek I, Beuthien-Baumann B, Ordemann R, et al. FDG PET/MR for the assessment of lymph node involvement in lymphoma: initial results and role of diffusion-weighted MR. Acad Radiol 2014;21(10): 1314–9.

33. Cerci JJ, Trindade E, Buccheri V, et al. Consistency of FDG-PET accuracy and cost-effectiveness in initial staging of patients with Hodgkin lymphoma across jurisdictions. Clin Lymphoma Myeloma Leuk 2011;11(4):314–20.

34. Hutchings M, Loft A, Hansen M, et al. Position emission tomography with or without computed tomography in the primary staging of Hodgkin's lymphoma. Haematologica 2006;91(4):482–9.

35. Heacock L, Weissbrot J, Raad R, et al. PET/MRI for the evaluation of patients with lymphoma: initial observations. AJR Am J Roentgenol 2015;204(4):842–8.

36. Littooij AS, Kwee TC, de Keizer B, et al. Whole-body MRI-DWI for assessment of residual disease after completion of therapy in lymphoma: a prospective multicenter study. J Magn Reson Imaging 2015; 42(6):1646–55.

37. Shields AF, Grierson JR, Dohmen BM, et al. Imaging proliferation in vivo with [F-18]FLT and positron emission tomography. Nat Med 1998;4(11):1334–6.

38. Lee H, Kim SK, Kim YI, et al. Early determination of prognosis by interim 3'-deoxy-3'-18F-fluorothymidine PET in patients with non-Hodgkin lymphoma. J Nucl Med 2014;55(2):216–22.

39. Graf N, Herrmann K, Numberger B, et al. [18F]FLT is superior to [18F]FDG for predicting early response to antiproliferative treatment in high-grade lymphoma in a dose-dependent manner. Eur J Nucl Med Mol Imaging 2012;40(1):34–43.

18F-Fluorodeoxyglucose PET/MR Imaging in Head and Neck Cancer

Ivan Platzek, MD

KEYWORDS

- PET/MRI • FDG • Head and neck cancer • Staging • Recurrence

KEY POINTS

- In patients with head and neck squamous cell carcinoma (HNSCC), FDG PET/MR imaging does not improve lymph node metastases detection in comparison with MR imaging.
- Detection of local recurrence in HNSCC is not improved when FDG PET/MR imaging is used. FDG PET/MR imaging has a higher sensitivity for HNSCC recurrence.
- The role of FDG PET/MR imaging for other indications such as detection of distant metastases or radiotherapy planning has yet to be evaluated.

INTRODUCTION

> - MR imaging and computed tomography (CT) are currently the most widely used modalities in head and neck imaging.
> - The main shortcomings of both methods are low accuracy for cervical lymph node metastases and suspected tumor recurrence.
> - FDG PET/CT helps to improve tumor recurrence detection, although its value for initial staging is disputed.
> - PET/MR imaging allows for a combination of high soft tissue contrast and molecular information, which is very promising in oncologic imaging.

This article reviews the use of PET/MR imaging in patients with malignancies of the head and neck region. Tumors of the head and neck region are among the 10 most common cancers worldwide.[1] Head and neck squamous cell carcinoma (HNSCC) accounts for the vast majority of malignancies of the head and neck.[2] The most important risk factors for HNSCC are alcohol use and smoking.[3] In recent years, human papilloma virus[4] and Epstein-Barr virus[5] have been identified as further risk factors. Exposure to ultraviolet light is an important risk factor for squamous cell carcinoma of the lips.[6]

Patients with malignancies of the head and neck region present with varying clinical symptoms, which depend on the size and location of the primary tumor and the presence of metastases. Common symptoms and signs include swelling, pain, dysphagia, epistaxis, hoarseness, and loosening of teeth. The first step in the evaluation of a patient with suspected head and neck malignancy is clinical examination. Beside inspection of the face, nasal cavity, oral cavity, and neck, clinical examination also includes palpation of the neck. Because HNSCC often spreads to cervical lymph nodes, in some patients a cervical lump is the first clinical sign of disease. The clinical examination is usually complemented by fiberoptic endoscopy. If a lesion is detected during endoscopy, an endoscopic biopsy is usually performed.

The author has nothing to disclose.
Department of Radiology, Dresden University Hospital, Fetscherstr. 74, Dresden 01307, Germany
E-mail address: ivan.platzek@uniklinikum-dresden.de

PET Clin 11 (2016) 375–386
http://dx.doi.org/10.1016/j.cpet.2016.05.002
1556-8598/16/$ – see front matter © 2016 Elsevier Inc. All rights reserved.

Fine needle aspiration can be used to acquire small tissue samples from neck masses not accessible by endoscopic biopsy, such as suspected lymph node metastases.[7]

ROLE OF IMAGING AND STAGING CLASSIFICATIONS

Although the final diagnosis of HNSCC is based on biopsy, imaging is also an indispensable part of HNSCC evaluation and a prerequisite for adequate therapy. In patients undergoing primary staging, imaging is usually performed after a biopsy is obtained.

The purpose of imaging in patients with newly diagnosed head and neck cancer is to assess the extent of the primary tumor and the extent and location of metastatic disease. Imaging is also used to plan radiation therapy, which is widely used in HNSCC patients who are not suitable for surgical treatment. In patients already treated for head and neck cancer, imaging is used to exclude local recurrence or metastatic disease.

Radiologists evaluating examinations of the head and neck region should be familiar with classifications used in initial staging of HNSCC, strengths and weaknesses of imaging methods, and possible imaging pitfalls that may be encountered.

The TNM system is used to describe the extent of the primary tumor and metastatic disease in HNSCC. Depending on the location of the primary tumor, the classification of T stage differs, whereas the definitions of N and M stage are identical regardless of the tumor location.[8] Cervical lymph node metastases are common in patients with HNSCC and are also a very important prognostic factor.[9] The location of cervical lymph nodes is usually described according to a classification introduced by the American Academy Committee for Head and Neck Surgery and Oncology,[10] which subdivides each neck side into 8 lymph node levels.

IMAGING METHODS

Currently, MR imaging and CT are the most widely used modalities for imaging of HNSCC. The choice between CT and MR imaging is influenced by availability, tumor location, the ability of the patient to tolerate an MR imaging examination, and the preference of the radiologists involved. PET/CT, the first hybrid modality available in clinical settings, is also often used.

COMPUTED TOMOGRAPHY

The main advantages of CT are wide availability, high spatial resolution, very short acquisition times, and relatively low cost. Furthermore, CT is well-suited for the evaluation of bony structures, which may be infiltrated by the tumor. Owing to continuing improvements of scanner hardware, CT has remained competitive with MR imaging for head and neck imaging. Modern CT scanners allow for the acquisition of isotropic datasets and thus multiplanar reconstruction. As the soft tissue contrast of nonenhanced CT is low, CT of the head and neck is usually performed with iodinated contrast media.

MR IMAGING

The main advantage of MR imaging relative to CT is its excellent soft tissue contrast. It allows for better assessment of local tumor spread and invasiveness than CT or PET/CT. The in-plane resolution of MR imaging is comparable with that of CT, although the slice thickness is typically greater. Gadolinium-based contrast agents are routinely used for MR imaging staging of HNSCC. In contrast with CT, MR imaging examinations are not associated with radiation exposure. However, the value of this advantage in patients with cancer who often undergo radiotherapy is questionable. Acquisition times for MR imaging are substantially longer compared with CT, and because of this MR imaging is more prone to motion artifacts. MR imaging is especially preferred in imaging of lesions of the oral cavity and the pharynx.[11,12] A common problem for both MR imaging and CT is their relatively low accuracy for detection of lymph node metastases, which is owing to the reliance of both methods on morphologic criteria for lymph node evaluation.[13,14]

ULTRASONOGRAPHY

Owing to its high spatial resolution, wide availability, and low cost, ultrasonography is widely used for the evaluation of lymph nodes. Ultrasonography has a high accuracy for detecting cervical lymph node metastases in patients with HNSCC.[15] However, it does not allow for evaluation of primary tumors of the head and neck region, and thus cannot be an equivalent alternative to MR imaging or CT for comprehensive staging of HNSCC.

PET/COMPUTED TOMOGRAPHY

Most squamous cell carcinoma and their metastases show a strong uptake of ^{18}F-fluorodeoxyglucose (FDG), which is the most widely used PET radiotracer in clinical practice and is also the preferred radiotracer for HNSCC imaging.

The role of FDG PET/CT in patients with HNSCC is still a matter of discussion; several studies have produced conflicting results regarding possible advantages of PET/CT, especially in initial staging. For example, Branstetter and colleagues[16] found that FDG PET/CT is superior to CT for detection of malignant lesions in patients with HNSCC. Similarly, Park and colleagues[17] have shown that FDG PET/CT improves detection of cervical lymph node metastases when compared with CT and MR imaging. In contrast, Seitz and colleagues[18] found no advantage for FDG PET/CT over MR imaging for initial staging of HNSCC. FDG PET/CT can help exclude second primary tumors, which occur in up to 10% of patients with HNSCC.[19]

Currently, FDG PET/CT cannot be recommended for routine initial HNSCC staging. However, FDG PET/CT has important advantages for other indications related to HNSCC. For example, FDG PET/CT significantly improves accuracy for detection of recurrent HNSCC in comparison with contrast-enhanced CT.[20] FDG PET/CT also is also very helpful for assessment of the head and neck after chemoradiotherapy owing to its high specificity and negative predictive value.[21] In patients with cervical lymph node metastasis from a carcinoma of unknown origin, FDG PET and FDG PET/CT help to detect the primary tumor.[22,23]

In addition, FDG PET/CT is increasingly used for radiation treatment planning in HNSCC.[24,25] In this case, the metabolic information provided by PET is helpful for target volume delineation, whereas CT data allow for the calculation of radiation dose distribution.

PET/MR IMAGING
Introduction and Rationale of PET/MR Imaging

Whole-body PET/MR imaging systems first became available in 2010, approximately a decade after PET/CT. A major reason for the relatively late introduction of PET/MR imaging are technical challenges related to the use of PET detectors in high magnetic fields, and also to MR-based attenuation correction for PET data. PET/MR imaging was not intended as a replacement of the already established PET/CT in general, but rather for use in applications in which both soft tissue contrast and tissue metabolism are of primary importance. At the time of the introduction of PET/MR imaging, imaging of HNSCC was assumed to be a very promising application for the new hybrid imaging modality, which combines the excellent soft tissue contrast of MR imaging and the metabolic information offered by PET.

PET/MR Imaging Technique

PET/MR imaging examinations consist of a fast MR imaging scan used for PET attenuation correction (attenuation MR imaging), a PET scan, and usually diagnostic MR imaging. In head and neck PET/MR imaging, diagnostic MR imaging is indispensable, because the resolution of attenuation MR imaging is not sufficient for adequate assessment of the complex neck anatomy. Whereas in sequential PET/MR imaging (historically the first type of PET/MR imaging allowing whole-body examinations) PET and MR imaging are performed one after the other, current systems allow for simultaneous PET and MR imaging acquisition and can thus reduce total acquisition times. Time-of-flight PET has also become available in simultaneous PET/MR imaging systems. The spatial resolution and sensitivity of PET detectors used in PET/MR imaging is closely comparable with the same parameters in contemporary PET/CT.

Owing to previous experience with FDG PET/CT, nearly all available studies about PET/MR imaging in HNSCC have used FDG as the radiotracer. As with PET and PET/CT scanning, the radiotracer is applied intravenously about 60 minutes before the start of the PET scan. The patients should fast for 4 to 6 hours before FDG injection. At the author's institution, patients undergoing FDG PET/MR imaging are injected with 4.5 MBq FDG/kg body weight.[26] To exclude synchronous tumors or distant metastases, the PET scan should cover the area from the skull base to the upper thighs.

The use of a surface coil is mandatory in PET/MR imaging of the head and neck given the small size of the anatomic structures to be imaged and the resultant need for high spatial resolution. Currently, MR imaging sequences used for head and neck imaging are identical to those used in conventional MR imaging of the same region. A routine MR imaging examination of the head and neck region includes T1-weighted turbo spin echo (TSE) images in transverse orientation, short tau inversion recovery TSE images in transverse and coronal orientations, and fat-suppressed contrast-enhanced T1-weighted TSE in transverse and coronal orientations. At the author's institution, a slice thickness of 3 mm with no interslice gap is used routinely in head and neck MR imaging. In our experience, this slice thickness represents a good compromise between spatial resolution and acquisition time. The sequences described cover the area between the skull base and the aortic arch. The suggested protocol for diagnostic MR imaging of the head and neck is summarized in **Table 1**.

The use of gadolinium-based contrast agents in FDG PET/MR imaging of the head and neck was initially justified by previous experience with standalone MR imaging. Kuhn and colleagues[27] were able to confirm that the addition of

Table 1
Suggested diagnostic MR imaging sequences for ^{18}F-fluorodeoxyglucose PET/MR imaging of the head and neck region

Sequence Type	Contrast-Enhanced	Orientation	Slice Thickness (mm)
T1 TSE	No	Axial	3
STIR TSE	No	Axial	3
STIR TSE	No	Coronal	3
T1 TSE FS	Yes	Axial	3
T1 TSE FS	Yes	Coronal	3

Abbreviations: FS, fat suppression; STIR, short tau inversion recovery; TSE, turbo spin echo.

contrast-enhanced images to FDG PET/MR imaging improves tumor delineation and assessment of tumor infiltration of adjacent structures.

In the last decade, there has been a lot of interest in extracranial applications of diffusion-weighted MR imaging (DWI), including the use of DWI for lymph node staging in HNSCC. Initial results obtained at a field strength of 1.5 T have been encouraging.[28] However, a recent study by Queiroz and colleagues[29] found that the addition of DWI does not improve the accuracy of FDG PET/MR imaging in patients with HNSCC. Furthermore, single-shot echo planar imaging sequences used in DWI are prone to susceptibility artifacts, which tend to occur at tissue–gas interfaces and are more pronounced at 3 T when compared with 1.5 T.[30] Because all currently available PET/MR imaging systems are equipped with 3-T main magnets, this is a further argument against the use of single-shot echo planar imaging DWI in FDG PET/MR imaging of HNSCC.

As mentioned, excluding synchronous tumors or distant metastases is important in HNSCC imaging. At our institution, the area between the aortic arch and the upper thighs is only covered by attenuation MR imaging, and diagnostic sequences are added only if the PET scan shows suspicious findings. The added value of diagnostic MR imaging outside of the neck has not been evaluated in HNSCC PET/MR imaging. However, in more modern simultaneous PET/MR imaging systems, the addition of some basic diagnostic MR imaging outside the neck will lead to no or little additional acquisition time and is worth considering.

Image Quality and Uptake Quantification in ^{18}F-fluorodeoxyglucose PET/MR Imaging

Some early studies after the introduction of whole-body PET/MR imaging were able to show that FDG PET/MR imaging is feasible for HNSCC imaging, with image quality equivalent to conventional PET or MR imaging.[31,32] Another study has also shown that PET image quality in FDG PET/MR imaging of the head and neck is equivalent to PET image quality in PET/CT.[33] These results are in line with multiple feasibility studies of FDG PET/MR imaging in other anatomic regions.

Although quantification of FDG uptake based on PET/MR imaging is possible, comparison of quantitative data between different scanner types (ie, PET/MR imaging and PET/CT) is problematic. This is partly owing to the inevitable time interval between such examinations in comparison studies. Available studies show higher maximum standardized uptake value for the modality (PET/MR imaging or PET/CT) performed at a later time point,[31,33] which can be attributed partly to an increase of tumor FDG uptake with time.

Imaging Findings

Imaging features of primary tumors and metastases in PET/MR imaging are identical to those known from the standalone imaging modalities. HNSCC usually presents as a mass, which is isointense to muscle on unenhanced T1-weighted images and hyperintense to muscle on short tau inversion recovery images or other fat-suppressed T2-weighted images (**Fig. 1**). The tumors mostly show strong gadolinium enhancement, although larger tumors may include nonenhancing necrotic areas. As in standalone PET or PET/CT, HNSCC has strong FDG uptake when compared with surrounding tissue or the salivary glands.

Lymph node metastases of HNSCC also show high FDG uptake, except for necrotic metastases in which uptake is found only in the remaining vital tissue. MR imaging criteria for malignancy in cervical lymph nodes include a maximum short diameter greater than 10 mm, necrosis, irregular margins, spherical shape, and lack of a fatty hilum.

Because PET/MR imaging is a hybrid imaging modality, differentiation between benign and malignant findings is based on the combined, and sometimes conflicting, PET and MR imaging findings. Because of this, it is important that reading of PET/MR imaging examinations is undertaken jointly by a nuclear medicine physician and a radiologist, or by a physician certified for both specialties.

Beside HNSCC and lymph node metastases, differential diagnoses for cervical masses include a number of malignant and benign lesions. For example, cervical lymph node enlargement can be a sign of nodal involvement in lymphoma or can be caused by reactive lymphadenopathy. Thyroglossal duct cysts or branchial cleft cysts can be mistaken for necrotic metastases. Furthermore,

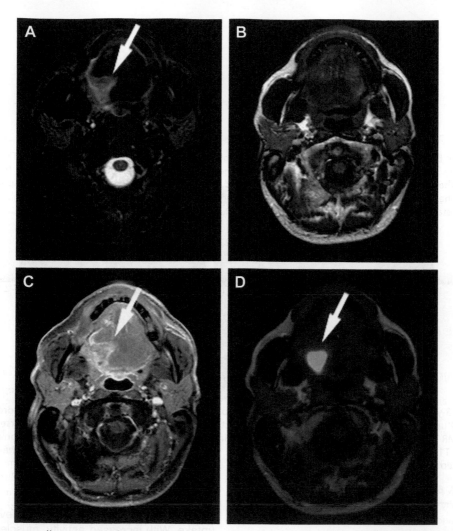

Fig. 1. Squamous cell carcinoma of right half of tongue. The tumor (*arrow*) is hyperintense compared with muscle in short tau inversion recovery image (*A*) and displays strong enhancement on contrast-enhanced T1-weighted image with fat suppression (*B*). On nonenhanced T1-weighted image, it is nearly isointense to muscle (*C*). It also shows strong ^{18}F-fluorodeoxyglucose (FDG) uptake, as shown on the combined axial FDG PET/MR image (*D*).

thyroid masses, glomus tumors, or schwannomas can also be mistaken for metastases.

Reactive cervical lymphadenopathy is especially difficult to differentiate from nodal metastatic disease, because reactive lymph nodes can be both enlarged and FDG avid. Other examples of benign lesions with high FDG uptake include pleomorphic adenoma of the salivary glands and Warthin tumor. Giant cell tumors, which are mostly benign (and locally invasive) but can also be malignant, also exhibit high FDG uptake (**Fig. 2**). Schwannoma can also display an increased FDG uptake, but have mostly more homogenous enhancement when compared with lymph nodes. Congenital cysts can sometimes be differentiated from necrotic metastases by their complete lack of solid enhancing components.

Important differential diagnoses for neck masses include:

- HNSCC,
- HNSCC nodal metastases,
- Reactive lymphadenopathy,
- Thyroid masses,
- Pleomorphic adenoma,
- Glomus tumor,
- Schwannoma,
- Thyroglossal duct cyst, and
- Branchial cleft cyst.

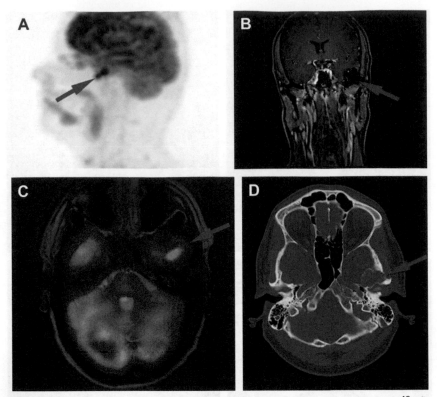

Fig. 2. A 33-year-old man with giant cell tumor (*arrow*) of left temporal bone showing high ^{18}F-fluorodeoxyglucose (FDG) uptake on sagittal maximum intensity projection (MIP) FDG PET image (*A*) and transverse combined FDG PET/MR image (*C*). The tumor has very low signal intensity on MR images, as shown on coronal contrast-enhanced T1-weighted image with fat suppression (*B*). The transverse computed tomography image demonstrates osteolysis by the lesion (*D*).

Pitfalls in PET/MR imaging

> *The most important pitfalls in FDG PET/MR imaging of the head and neck include:*
>
> - Muscle activation,
> - Metal artifacts,
> - Hypoglossal nerve palsy, and
> - Brown fat.

Although FDG uptake in HNSCC and HNSCC metastases is clearly increased in most cases, FDG is not a tumor-specific radiotracer. Increased FDG uptake in benign processes may be misinterpreted as malignant lesions. In addition, MR imaging is prone to susceptibility artifacts, which can be caused by dental implants and may obscure both anatomic structures and malignant findings, for example. The most relevant pitfalls in FDG PET/MR imaging of the head and neck are summarized below.

MUSCLE ACTIVATION

Resting muscles usually have a low level of FDG uptake. With increased activity, muscles increasingly use glucose as an energy source, and thus muscle contraction leads to stronger FDG uptake. Because of this, patients are advised to relax, remain seated or reclined, and refrain from major movement after FDG injection. Despite such precautions, increased FDG uptake is sometimes seen in neck muscles and/or laryngeal muscles (**Fig. 3**) or extraocular eye muscles, which can lead to false-positive findings. Careful comparison with MR imaging and multiplanar reconstruction of PET data help to differentiate between intramuscular and extramuscular radiotracer uptake. Furthermore, muscle FDG uptake is mostly linear in configuration, in contrast with the more focal or irregular uptake seen in malignant lesions.

METAL ARTIFACTS

Susceptibility artifacts are a significant problem in MR imaging and PET/MR imaging of the head and neck owing to the high percentage of patients

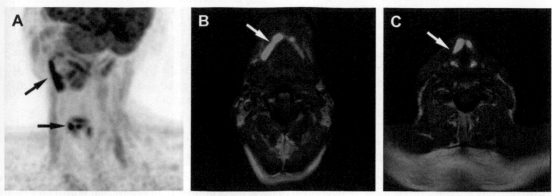

Fig. 3. A 64-year-old man with increased bilateral ^{18}F-fluorodeoxyglucose (FDG) uptake (*black arrows*) in cervical muscles and laryngeal muscles on oblique coronal maximum intensity projection FDG PET image (*A*). Transverse combined FDG PET/MR images demonstrate FDG uptake (*white arrows*) located in anterior bellies of digastric muscle (*B*) and laryngeal muscles (*C*).

with dental implants. The artifacts manifest as areas of signal void combined with image distortion. TSE sequences, the most widely used sequence type in head and neck MR imaging, are less prone to such artifacts than gradient recalled echo sequences or EPI sequences. However, susceptibility artifacts can obscure even comparatively large lesions, depending on location (**Fig. 4**). In such cases, PET and MR imaging are truly complimentary, because PET image quality is much less influenced by metallic objects when compared with MR imaging. In addition, in our experience, MR imaging-based attenuation correction in PET/MR imaging of the head and neck is effective in currently available systems despite the susceptibility artifacts.

HYPOGLOSSAL NERVE PALSY

Contralateral hypoglossal nerve palsy causes 1-sided atrophy of the tongue muscles. The asymmetry of the tongue muscles can lead to asymmetric FDG uptake of the tongue, which can be mistaken for a tumor. Careful review of the tongue on MR images usually helps to identify muscle atrophy and explain tongue radiotracer uptake asymmetry.

BROWN FAT

In adults, brown fat is found mostly in the lower neck and upper mediastinum. It can show increased FDG uptake, especially in patients with low body fat and in cold weather. The increased FDG uptake of brown adipose tissue is mostly symmetrical, and coregistration with MR images in most cases allows one to differentiate this benign finding from metastatic disease (**Fig. 5**). In cases with inconclusive findings, FDG uptake in brown adipose fat can be reduced by administering beta-blockers.

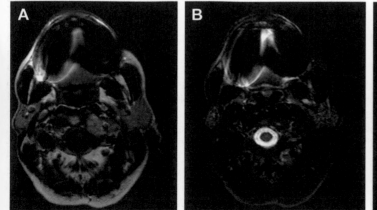
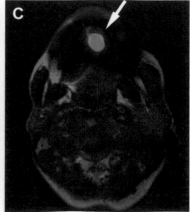

Fig. 4. A 55-year-old man with squamous cell carcinoma of tongue. Owing to susceptibility artifacts, the tumor is obscured on transverse T1-weighted imaging (*A*) and transverse short tau inversion recovery imaging (*B*). In contrast, tumor (*arrow*) is well-visualized on transverse combined ^{18}F-fluorodeoxyglucose PET/MR image (*C*), because PET is much less influenced by metal implants.

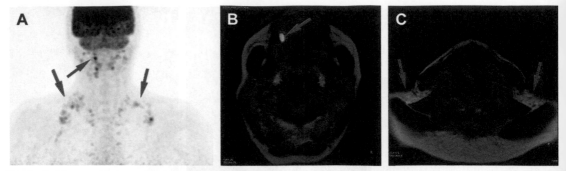

Fig. 5. A 55-year-old woman undergoing staging evaluation for head and neck squamous cell carcinoma with brown fat. Note increased symmetrical ^{18}F-fluorodeoxyglucose (FDG) uptake in supraclavicular brown fat (*red arrows*) on coronal maximum intensity projection (MIP) FDG PET imaging (*A*) and transverse combined PET/MR imaging (*C*). Also note stronger and more localized FDG uptake (*blue arrows*) in squamous cell carcinoma of tongue as seen on coronal MIP FDG PET imaging (*A*) and transverse combined PET/MR imaging (*B*).

^{18}F-FLUORODEOXYGLUCOSE PET/MR IMAGING OF THE HEAD AND NECK COMPARED WITH OTHER IMAGING METHODS

After the feasibility of PET/MR imaging of the head and neck was established by early studies, later projects sought to compare PET/MR imaging to other imaging modalities and establish its role in management of HNSCC. Currently, a number of comparison studies on PET/MR imaging in HNSCC are available, including studies focusing on initial staging and on detection of suspected tumor recurrence, although multicentric studies are still lacking.

INITIAL STAGING

FDG PET/MR imaging is superior to standalone MR imaging (**Fig. 6**) for primary tumor detection.[34] At first glance, this advantage is questionable

because the location of the primary tumor is usually already known from clinical examination or endoscopy. Increased confidence about tumor thickness owing to improved tumor visualization with PET/MR imaging may be useful for planning of surgical therapy. Until now, tumor thickness estimations based on PET/MR imaging have not been compared with histologically verified tumor thickness.

As mentioned, cervical lymph node metastases are one of the most important prognostic factors in HNSCC. PET can help to identify normal sized metastatic lymph nodes that are not detectable with MR imaging (**Fig. 7**). Also, MR imaging can depict necrotic lymph node metastases that may otherwise be missed by PET (**Fig. 8**). Yet, false positives and micrometastases still present a diagnostic challenge. Studies that have investigated initial staging in HNSCC found no significant advantage of FDG PET/MR imaging over standalone MR imaging or standalone PET with regard

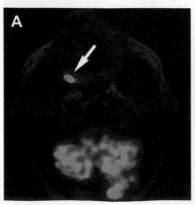
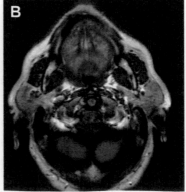
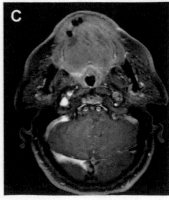

Fig. 6. A 70-year-old man with a tumor of the right palatoglossal arch. The tumor (*arrow*) is well-visualized on transverse combined ^{18}F-fluorodeoxyglucose PET/MR imaging (*A*), but is not visible on transverse T1-weighted MR imaging (*B*) or on transverse contrast-enhanced T1-weighted image with fat suppression (*C*).

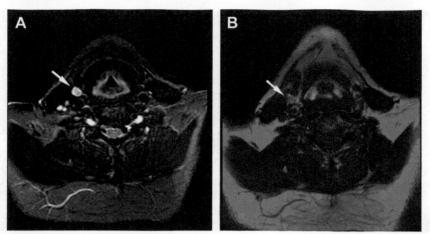

Fig. 7. A 64-year-old man with metastatic lymph node (*arrow*). The metastasis was detected on transverse combined ^{18}F-fluorodeoxyglucose (FDG) PET/MR imaging (*B*) owing to its high FDG uptake, but not on standalone MR imaging. The transverse short tau inversion recovery MR imaging (*A*) demonstrates that right cervical metastatic lymph node is not enlarged (maximum largest transverse diameter of 8 mm).

to accuracy for detection of cervical lymph node metastases.[34,35] In summary, there is currently no justification for the use of FDG PET/MR imaging instead of MR imaging for primary staging of HNSCC.

FOLLOW-UP

Although the normal anatomy of the neck is already complex, the neck of a patient who has already underwent treatment for HNSCC is even more of a challenge for the radiologist and the nuclear medicine physician. In such patients, scar tissue and resulting asymmetry make the

detection of recurrent tumors difficult, as does possible increased FDG uptake that may occur in tissue inflamed owing to chemoradiation or recent surgery. Recurrent tumors (**Fig. 9**) most often have greater FDG uptake than inflamed tissue, but nevertheless small lesions may be difficult to recognize.

Queiroz and colleagues[36] compared FDG PET/MR imaging with MR imaging and PET/CT in patients with suspected HNSCC recurrence to evaluate possible advantages of the new hybrid modality. Although the authors found PET/MR imaging to be more useful than PET/CT in several cases with ambiguous FDG uptake findings, the

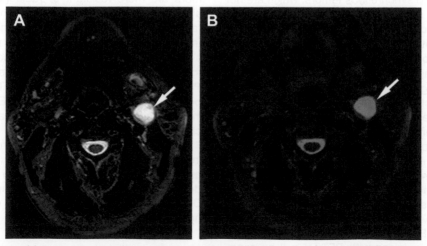

Fig. 8. A 60-year-old man with necrotic metastatic lymph node (*arrow*). The transverse short tau inversion recovery MR image (*A*) shows enlarged left cervical lymph node with very high signal intensity owing to necrosis. The corresponding transverse combined ^{18}F-fluorodeoxyglucose (FDG) PET/MR image (*B*) shows very little FDG uptake in metastasis owing to extensive necrosis.

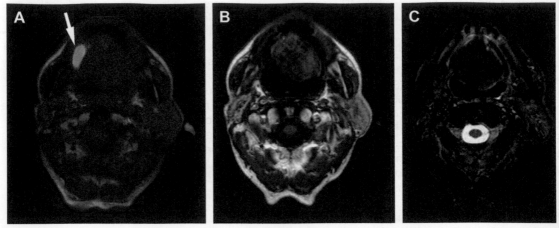

Fig. 9. A 78-year-old man with recurrent tumor of right floor of mouth. The tumor recurrence (*arrow*) is visible on transverse combined ^{18}F-fluorodeoxyglucose (FDG) PET/MR imaging (*A*) given its high FDG uptake, but was not detected on standalone MR imaging as demonstrated on transverse T1-weighted imaging (*B*) and transverse short tau inversion recovery imaging (*C*).

diagnostic accuracy of PET/MR imaging and PET/CT did not differ significantly. The sensitivity of FDG PET/MR Imaging was higher than the sensitivity of MR imaging, whereas the specificity of both methods was very similar.

DISTANT METASTASES, SYNCHRONOUS TUMORS, AND CARCINOMA OF UNKNOWN PRIMARY

Because distant metastases are less common than nodal metastases in patients referred for initial staging of HNSCC, a systematic evaluation of the role of PET/MR imaging for systematic metastases is not available currently. The same is true with regard to synchronous tumors, which are not uncommon in patients with HNSCC[37] and are mostly found in the upper aerodigestive tract or the lung. With regard to both distant metastases and synchronous tumors, the accuracy of FDG PET/MR imaging for lung lesions is especially relevant. Although MR imaging is still clearly inferior to CT for detection of small lung lesions, detection of pulmonary lesions larger than 8 to 10 mm is usually not a problem with modern MR imaging systems. A relatively recent study of patients with different primary tumors have shown that the detection rate of pulmonary metastases is lower for FDG PET/MR imaging than that for FDG PET/CT.[38]

In patients with neck metastases of unknown primary or with carcinoma of unknown primary, the role of PET/MR imaging has not yet been evaluated. A comparison with PET/CT will be especially important in this context, because occult HNSCC is mostly detected owing to increased FDG uptake whereas the anatomic component of the hybrid imaging (CT vs MR imaging) is expected to be of secondary importance.

The role of PET/MR imaging in patients with tumors other than HNSCC in the head and neck region has also yet to be evaluated systematically.

ALTERNATIVE RADIOTRACERS

All radiotracers used in PET and PET/CT can be used in PET/MR imaging. Because nearly all HNSCCs are FDG avid, the use of alternative radiotracers in head and neck imaging has been sporadic. With PET/CT, there have been several studies using ^{18}F-fluoromisonidazole for the evaluation of tumor hypoxia in HNSCC.[39,40] Hypoxic tumors are more resistant to radiochemotherapy, and thus hypoxia imaging is of prognostic importance and also potentially of importance for radiotherapy planning. Hypoxia imaging is not currently a part of clinical practice and is focused mostly on the PET component. Because of this, the use of PET/MR imaging instead of PET/CT is not expected to bring major benefits. No PET/MR imaging studies using ^{18}F-fluoromisonidazole in this clinical setting have been reported.

An interesting possible application of PET/MR imaging in the head and neck is for imaging assessment of glomus tumors. One case report describes the use of PET/MR imaging with ^{68}Ga-DOTATATE,[41] although a systematic evaluation is not currently available.

SUMMARY

FDG PET/MR imaging does not offer a significant advantage over MR imaging for initial staging of

HNSCC. With all imaging modalities, detection of cervical lymph node metastases remains a challenge in head and neck imaging. With currently available radiotracers and MR imaging techniques, it is unlikely that PET/MR imaging will contribute significantly to the solution of this problem. In patients with suspected recurrence of HNSCC, PET/MR imaging has higher sensitivity than MR imaging, but does not improve accuracy compared with FDG PET/CT. It remains to be seen if the improved depiction of anatomy with PET/MR imaging will have an impact on the choice of therapy in HNSCC recurrence when compared with PET/CT.

What the referring physician needs to know:

- FDG PET/MR imaging is a new hybrid imaging modality which allows for a comprehensive staging of head and neck cancer.

- Currently, FDG PET/MR imaging cannot be recommended for initial staging of HNSCC, because it does not show significant advantages over the less expensive and much more widespread MR imaging in available studies.

- In patients with suspected HNSCC recurrence, FDG PET/MR imaging is superior to stand-alone MR imaging. The added value of FDG PET/MR imaging in comparison with FDG PET/CT in suspected recurrence has yet to be clarified.

REFERENCES

1. Jemal A, Bray F, Center MM, et al. Global cancer statistics. CA Cancer J Clin 2011;61(2):69–90.

2. Curado MP, Hashibe M. Recent changes in the epidemiology of head and neck cancer. Curr Opin Oncol 2009;21(3):194–200.

3. Lubin JH, Purdue M, Kelsey K, et al. Total exposure and exposure rate effects for alcohol and smoking and risk of head and neck cancer: a pooled analysis of case-control studies. Am J Epidemiol 2009; 170(8):937–47.

4. Mork J, Lie AK, Glattre E, et al. Human papillomavirus infection as a risk factor for squamous-cell carcinoma of the head and neck. N Engl J Med 2001; 344(15):1125–31.

5. Gillison ML, Koch WM, Capone RB, et al. Evidence for a causal association between human papillomavirus and a subset of head and neck cancers. J Natl Cancer Inst 2000;92(9):709–20.

6. Perea-Milla Lopez E, Minarro-Del Moral RM, Martinez-Garcia C, et al. Lifestyles, environmental and phenotypic factors associated with lip cancer: a case-control study in southern Spain. Br J Cancer 2003;88(11):1702–7.

7. el Hag IA, Chiedozi LC, al Reyees FA, et al. Fine needle aspiration cytology of head and neck masses. Seven years' experience in a secondary care hospital. Acta Cytol 2003;47(3):387–92.

8. Wittekind C, Asamura H, Sobin LH, editors. TNM atlas. 6th edition. Chichester (United Kingdom); West Sussex (United Kingdom): Wiley Blackwell; 2014.

9. Mamelle G, Pampurik J, Luboinski B, et al. Lymph node prognostic factors in head and neck squamous cell carcinomas. Am J Surg 1994;168(5): 494–8.

10. Robbins KT, Medina JE, Wolfe GT, et al. Standardizing neck dissection terminology. Official report of the Academy's Committee for Head and Neck Surgery and Oncology. Arch Otolaryngol Head Neck Surg 1991;117(6):601–5.

11. Ong CK, Chong VF. Imaging of tongue carcinoma. Cancer Imaging 2006;6:186–93.

12. Kosling S, Knipping S, Hofmockel T. Imaging of nasopharyngeal diseases. HNO 2009;57(8):813–24 [quiz: 825]. [in German].

13. Castelijns JA, van den Brekel MW. Detection of lymph node metastases in the neck: radiologic criteria. AJNR Am J Neuroradiol 2001;22(1):3–4.

14. van den Brekel MW, Stel HV, Castelijns JA, et al. Cervical lymph node metastasis: assessment of radiologic criteria. Radiology 1990;177(2):379–84.

15. de Bondt RBJ, Nelemans PJ, Hofman PAM, et al. Detection of lymph node metastases in head and neck cancer: a meta-analysis comparing US, USgFNAC, CT and MR imaging. Eur J Radiol 2007;64(2): 266–72.

16. Branstetter BF 4th, Blodgett TM, Zimmer LA, et al. Head and neck malignancy: is PET/CT more accurate than PET or CT alone? Radiology 2005;235(2): 580–6.

17. Park JT, Roh JL, Kim JS, et al. 18F FDG PET/CT versus CT/MR imaging and the prognostic value of contralateral neck metastasis in patients with head and neck squamous cell carcinoma. Radiology 2016;279(2):481–91.

18. Seitz O, Chambron-Pinho N, Middendorp M, et al. 18F-Fluorodeoxyglucose-PET/CT to evaluate tumor, nodal disease, and gross tumor volume of oropharyngeal and oral cavity cancer: comparison with MR imaging and validation with surgical specimen. Neuroradiology 2009;51(10):677–86.

19. Strobel K, Haerle SK, Stoeckli SJ, et al. Head and neck squamous cell carcinoma (HNSCC) – detection of synchronous primaries with 18F-FDG-PET/CT. Eur J Nucl Med Mol Imaging 2009;36(6):919–27.

20. Suenaga Y, Kitajima K, Ishihara T, et al. FDG-PET/contrast-enhanced CT as a post-treatment tool in head and neck squamous cell carcinoma:

comparison with FDG-PET/non-contrast-enhanced CT and contrast-enhanced CT. Eur Radiol 2016; 26(4):1018–30.

21. Ong SC, Schoder H, Lee NY, et al. Clinical utility of 18F-FDG PET/CT in assessing the neck after concurrent chemoradiotherapy for Locoregional advanced head and neck cancer. J Nucl Med 2008;49(4):532–40.

22. Rusthoven KE, Koshy M, Paulino AC. The role of fluorodeoxyglucose positron emission tomography in cervical lymph node metastases from an unknown primary tumor. Cancer 2004;101(11):2641–9.

23. Johansen J, Eigtved A, Buchwald C, et al. Implication of 18F-fluoro-2-deoxy-D-glucose positron emission tomography on management of carcinoma of unknown primary in the head and neck: a Danish cohort study. Laryngoscope 2002;112(11):2009–14.

24. Gregoire V, Chiti A. Molecular imaging in radiotherapy planning for head and neck tumors. J Nucl Med 2011;52(3):331–4.

25. Schwartz DL, Ford EC, Rajendran J, et al. FDG-PET/CT-guided intensity modulated head and neck radiotherapy: a pilot investigation. Head Neck 2005;27(6):478–87.

26. Boellaard R, O'Doherty MJ, Weber WA, et al. FDG PET and PET/CT: EANM procedure guidelines for tumour PET imaging: version 1.0. Eur J Nucl Med Mol Imaging 2010;37(1):181–200.

27. Kuhn FP, Hullner M, Mader CE, et al. Contrast-enhanced PET/MR imaging versus contrast-enhanced PET/CT in head and neck cancer: how much MR information is needed? J Nucl Med 2014;55(4):551–8.

28. Holzapfel K, Duetsch S, Fauser C, et al. Value of diffusion-weighted MR imaging in the differentiation between benign and malignant cervical lymph nodes. Eur J Radiol 2009;72(3):381–7.

29. Queiroz MA, Hullner M, Kuhn F, et al. Use of diffusion-weighted imaging (DWI) in PET/MRI for head and neck cancer evaluation. Eur J Nucl Med Mol Imaging 2014;41(12):2212–21.

30. Mazaheri Y, Vargas HA, Nyman G, et al. Image artifacts on prostate diffusion-weighted magnetic resonance imaging: trade-offs at 1.5 Tesla and 3.0 Tesla. Acad Radiol 2013;20(8):1041–7.

31. Platzek I, Beuthien-Baumann B, Schneider M, et al. PET/MRI in head and neck cancer: initial experience. Eur J Nucl Med Mol Imaging 2013;40(1):6–11.

32. Abdulqadhr G, Molin D, Astrom G, et al. Whole-body diffusion-weighted imaging compared with FDG-PET/CT in staging of lymphoma patients. Acta Radiol 2011;52(2):173–80.

33. Varoquaux A, Rager O, Poncet A, et al. Detection and quantification of focal uptake in head and neck tumours: (18)F-FDG PET/MR versus PET/CT. Eur J Nucl Med Mol Imaging 2014;41(3):462–75.

34. Platzek I, Beuthien-Baumann B, Schneider M, et al. FDG PET/MR for lymph node staging in head and neck cancer. Eur J Radiol 2014;83(7):1163–8.

35. Kubiessa K, Purz S, Gawlitza M, et al. Initial clinical results of simultaneous 18F-FDG PET/MRI in comparison to 18F-FDG PET/CT in patients with head and neck cancer. Eur J Nucl Med Mol Imaging 2014;41(4):639–48.

36. Queiroz MA, Hullner M, Kuhn F, et al. PET/MRI and PET/CT in follow-up of head and neck cancer patients. Eur J Nucl Med Mol Imaging 2014;41(6):1066–75.

37. Nikolaou AC, Markou CD, Petridis DG, et al. Second primary neoplasms in patients with laryngeal carcinoma. Laryngoscope 2000;110(1):58–64.

38. Rauscher I, Eiber M, Furst S, et al. PET/MR imaging in the detection and characterization of pulmonary lesions: technical and diagnostic evaluation in comparison to PET/CT. J Nucl Med 2014;55(5):724–9.

39. Rajendran JG, Schwartz DL, O'Sullivan J, et al. Tumor hypoxia imaging with [F-18] fluoromisonidazole positron emission tomography in head and neck cancer. Clin Cancer Res 2006;12(18):5435–41.

40. Kikuchi M, Yamane T, Shinohara S, et al. 18F-fluoromisonidazole positron emission tomography before treatment is a predictor of radiotherapy outcome and survival prognosis in patients with head and neck squamous cell carcinoma. Ann Nucl Med 2011;25(9):625–33.

41. Beuthien-Baumann B, Platzek I, Lauterbach I, et al. Improved anatomic visualization of a glomus caroticum tumour within the carotic bifurcation with combined 68Ga-DOTATATE PET/MRI. Eur J Nucl Med Mol Imaging 2012;39(6):1087–8.

Clinical PET-MR Imaging in Breast Cancer and Lung Cancer

Samuel L. Rice, MD, Kent P. Friedman, MD*

KEYWORDS

- PET-MR imaging • Hybrid imaging • Breast cancer • Lung cancer • Oncology • Thoracic imaging

KEY POINTS

- PET-MR imaging may potentially detect more distant metastases in breast cancer compared with PET-CT or MR imaging alone, and it has the potential to guide breast biopsies based on higher specificity compared with MR imaging.
- PET-MR imaging has the potential to detect distant metastases of lung cancer with even higher sensitivity than PET-CT or MR imaging alone.
- Current PET-MR imaging systems will not replace chest computed tomography (CT) for detection of small primary lung tumors.
- PET-MR imaging offers advantages compared with PET-CT with respect to molecular-anatomic lesion registration, motion correction, radiation dose, and patient convenience.
- PET-MR imaging has the potential to allow precise quantification of molecular information obtained by both PET and MR imaging, and allows for voxelwise correlation and temporally aligned data that may inform patient management in the future.

INTRODUCTION

Advances in radiographic computed tomography (CT), MR imaging, PET, and combined PET-CT have dramatically improved the management of patients with cancer over the past 2 decades. For years, researchers and clinicians have wondered if combining PET with MR imaging would offer similar or even greater advantages compared with PET-CT.

Recent advancements in MR imaging scanners and the advent of MR imaging-compatible solid-state PET detectors that replace traditional photomultiplier tubes have made it possible to finally combine MR imaging and PET into a single device that acquires whole-body PET-MR images. Potential advantages of hybrid PET-MR imaging compared with PET-CT include superior identification of lesions in the brain, breast, liver, kidney, and bones, as well as enhanced evaluation of the margins of lesions. Improved anatomic registration with PET secondary to simultaneous image acquisition is now a reality with the advent of simultaneous PET-MR imaging scanners. Furthermore, the application of multiparametric quantitative imaging in MR imaging and functional PET has the potential to better guide patient management and to decrease the number of imaging studies required for clinical decision-making, resulting in less radiation exposure and improved patient satisfaction (**Box 1**).

Neoplasms of the thorax, including those of the breast and lung, are some of the most commonly

The authors have nothing to disclose.
Division of Nuclear Medicine, Department of Radiology, New York University Langone Medical Center, 660 First Avenue, New York, NY 10016, USA
* Corresponding author.
E-mail address: kent.friedman@nyumc.org

PET Clin 11 (2016) 387–402
http://dx.doi.org/10.1016/j.cpet.2016.05.008
1556-8598/16/$ – see front matter

pet.theclinics.com

Box 1
Typical breast cancer or lung cancer PET-MR imaging protocol

- 15 mCi ^{18}F- 2-fluoro-2-deoxy-D-glucose (FDG) intravenously, wait 60 minutes, void
  - Can perform diagnostic breast MR imaging during radiotracer uptake period if desired (for patients with breast cancer)
- Scan from skull vertex to thighs
- Multichannel head and neck coil, flexible body coil
- 6 minutes per bed PET acquisition with simultaneous MR imaging sequences
  - Dixon MR imaging attenuation correction images
  - 3-dimensional T1-weighted images
  - 3 b-value diffusion-weighted imaging (DWI)
  - Axial T2-weighted half-Fourier single-shot turbo spin echo (HASTE) or short tau inversion recovery (STIR) images if desired by imaging physician
- Inject gadolinium-based contrast material intravenously
  - Postcontrast 3-dimensional T1-weighted images of liver and brain

---

improved the potential molecular imaging capabilities of PET, accurately permitting in vivo imaging of various important clinical markers, including cell surface receptor expression, DNA production or repair, and hypoxia.[2,3] MR imaging has also evolved with new and faster sequences that allow for whole-body imaging, as well as functional imaging sequences, including magnetic resonance spectroscopy (MRS), perfusion imaging, and diffusion-weighted imaging (DWI), which have expanded the use of MR imaging in characterizing disease. With all of the added benefits of combined PET-MR imaging, the imaging algorithm currently used for thoracic cancers can be further optimized, potentially allowing for superior clinical information to be obtained from a single scan (**Box 2**).

PET-COMPUTED TOMOGRAPHY IN BREAST CANCER

Breast cancer remains exceedingly prevalent in the Western world and is a leading cause of mortality in women. Once diagnosed, survival is inversely related to the extent of disease at diagnosis, currently characterized with the tumor-node-metastasis (TNM) staging system. Metastases to axillary lymph nodes have a profound influence on patient prognosis, with

---

diagnosed cancers in the western world, which cause exceptionally high morbidity and mortality and are areas of active study in the emerging field of clinical PET-MR imaging. According to cancer statistics in 2015, approximately 234,190 people were diagnosed with breast cancer and 221,200 were diagnosed with lung neoplasms in the United States; this includes an estimated 40,730 and 158,040 related deaths secondary to these 2 diseases, respectively.[1] Overall survival is greatly influenced by the stage of the neoplasm at the time of diagnosis and by the histologic subtype of cancer.

PET systems have greatly improved in the last few decades with faster imaging time and improved scanner resolution; the combination of CT with hybrid PET-CT scanners has merged anatomic and molecular imaging, allowing for more accurate diagnosis and staging of many neoplasms. ^{18}F- 2-fluoro-2-deoxy-D-glucose (FDG) is a radioactive analogue of glucose and the most commonly used PET radiotracer in clinical practice. The clinical implementation of multiple novel clinical PET radiotracers, along with ongoing research of various others, has advanced and

---

Box 2
PET-MR imaging pitfalls in breast and lung cancers

- Metallic artifacts in breast tissue expanders can generate signal dropout on attenuation maps and result in underestimation of standardized uptake value (SUV) in chest wall lesions.
- Misclassification of lung tissue as air can underestimate SUV in lung lesions.
- Misclassification of hilar lymph nodes as air can result in SUV underestimation.
- Clinical PET-MR imaging readers should keep in mind the breath-hold protocol for various sequences obtained during PET-MR imaging and understand the potential for lesion misregistration relative to PET.
- MR imaging motion-tracking holds great promise for motion correction of PET datasets in the near future, without additional radiation exposure.
- Geometric distortion on DWI datasets results in misregistration to PET data; this should be kept in mind during clinical interpretation.

10-year survival ranging from 90% without the presence of lymphatic spread down to 30% when greater than 10 lymph nodes are involved.[4] Currently, the primary role of FDG PET-CT in patients with breast cancer is for assessment of suspected tumor recurrence or staging of locally advanced disease (ie, with large primary tumors >50 mm in size, chest wall tumor involvement, or axillary, internal mammary, or infraclavicular or supraclavicular lymph node metastases). Evidence exists that patients with inflammatory breast cancer also benefit from early FDG PET-CT imaging.[4–6]

Current guidelines for initial staging of breast cancer include physical examination, biopsy with histologic evaluation, and an array of imaging modalities, including mammography, ultrasonography, MR imaging, and potentially FDG PET-CT. The sensitivity of FDG PET-CT for small tumors less than 10 mm (T1 stage) has been shown to range from 50% to 72%, with the sensitivity of FDG PET-CT increasing to greater than 90% for tumors between 20 to 50 mm.[7–9] FDG PET-CT has been shown to underestimate the extent of disease within the breast when compared with MR imaging, with the accuracy of correctly diagnosing the degree of primary disease in the breast found to be 54% and 77%, respectively, for these 2 imaging modalities.[8,10,11] The poor performance of whole-body FDG PET-CT in evaluating primary tumors in the breast can be attributed to volume averaging due to the small size of the lesion, the generally lower hexokinase activity of breast cancer when compared with other cancer types, variations in tumor FDG uptake secondary to histologic subtype, and the background FDG uptake of normal breast tissue.[12–14] FDG PET-CT for the assessment of lymph node disease has a sensitivity, specificity, positive predictive value, and negative predictive value of 61%, 80%, 62%, and 79%, respectively.[15] This underestimation of the number of lymph nodes involved precludes it from replacing sentinel lymph node biopsy for primary evaluation of local spread and micrometastatic disease.

There has been extensive research in the use of changes in FDG uptake measured by standardized uptake value (SUV) within the tumor to assess for treatment response. Multiple studies have observed a statistically significant decrease in tumor FDG uptake in patients who have responded to therapy compared with those who have had no response. Evidence has also been presented that changes in SUV correlate with pathologic response to therapy.[16–19] Currently, clinicians use these changes to guide management decisions although determination of how to best leverage PET data in the setting of myriad cytostatic treatment options remains an area of active research (**Box 3**).

FDG PET-CT has also been validated for the accurate detection of recurrent breast cancer irrespective of histologic subtype with a sensitivity of 92% to 96% and a specificity of 75% to 90%.[19–22]

MR IMAGING IN BREAST CANCER

MR imaging is a highly utilized imaging modality for the evaluation of breast lesions in conjunction with mammography and ultrasonography. MR imaging is currently used and approved for a number purposes, including screening in women considered to be at high risk for disease (ie, lifetime risk >20%), assessment of patients with prior breast augmentation surgery, evaluation of the extent of disease in newly diagnosed patients (multifocal vs multicenter disease, chest wall invasion), and evaluation of response in patients who received neoadjuvant chemotherapy.[23,24]

Breast MR imaging typically uses a 1.5 or 3.0 T scanner; the patient is placed in the prone position with a dedicated breast coil used to acquire images with chemical fat suppression. Precontrast and postcontrast T1-weighted images are

---

Box 3
What the referring physician needs to know about PET-MR imaging

- PET-MR imaging performance is comparable to PET-CT in breast cancer and lung cancer.

- Preliminary evidence suggests a potential advantage of PET-MR imaging in detection or brain, bone marrow, liver, and adrenal gland metastases in breast cancer and lung cancer.

- Increased sensitivity in these organs comes at a cost of lower sensitivity for small lung metastases.

- PET-MR imaging examinations offer a convenient study for patients who require both PET and MR imaging, with reduced radiation exposure and potentially shorter total scan time compared with separate PET-CT and MR imaging.

- PET-MR imaging allows generation of multi-parametric quantitative datasets; preliminary research suggests possible synergy between SUV, DWI, and contrast-enhanced MR imaging parameters; however, future research is required before quantitative PET-MR imaging will directly influence patient management.

obtained using a gradient echo technique. Detection of neoplasms within the breast is primarily achieved by evaluating the dynamic contrast enhancement of a lesion in which the variable uptake kinetics of contrast material help to distinguish malignant from benign lesions.[25] Various other techniques have been used to improve the specificity of diagnosis, including the use of other imaging characteristics of a lesion. On MR imaging, the findings of rapid or medium initial contrast uptake (type II and III kinetic curves) or contrast washout on delayed phase images within lesions have a 77% positive predictive value for malignancy.[26–28] MR imaging is able to detect tumors at 10 mm, which is smaller than other commonly used imaging techniques.[29–31] MR imaging has also been shown to be highly sensitive but not specific, with a negative predictive value of 95% but a specificity of only 25%. A limitation of MR imaging of the breast includes normal cyclic changes in background breast tissue parenchymal enhancement by changing hormonal status of the patient, which limits its usefulness in younger patients but increases its specificity in postmenopausal women.[26–28]

Breast MR imaging can also be used to evaluate lymph node involvement by identifying an increase in size, increased contrast enhancement, and lack of a normal fatty hilum. MR imaging has a sensitivity and specificity of 90% and 82%, respectively, for the detection of metastatic disease in lymph nodes when using size greater than 5 mm and abnormally increased enhancement.[32] A limitation to evaluating lymph nodes in the axilla is that standard breast coils have inadequate coverage of the axilla. Whole-body MR imaging is not used regularly for the evaluation of systemic metastatic disease or distant tumor recurrence.

PET-MR IMAGING IN BREAST CANCER

The theoretical advantages of PET-MR imaging compared with PET-CT or MR imaging alone are just starting to be explored in preliminary clinical research. Much early work has focused on studies of technical feasibility and reproducibility of SUV quantification between PET-MR imaging and PET-CT. Early data are emerging that suggest a potential additive clinical value of PET-MR imaging and which may serve as the basis for larger studies. It is likely that to prove any further increase in diagnostic accuracy of PET-MR imaging compared with PET-CT, large multi-institutional trials will be required to assess for statistically significant incremental increases in sensitivity or specificity.

Many questions exist regarding quantitative differences with respect to SUV obtained from PET-CT and PET-MR imaging. Whereas CT-based attenuation correction directly measures attenuation throughout the body, current MR imaging-based attenuation correction algorithms use methods to segment tissues into basic categories, including fat, soft tissue, air, and lung parenchyma. Some newer techniques are emerging that seek to map the locations of bones. All of these techniques are based on fixed estimates of tissue density that may or may not reflect the clinical reality for individual patients. Lung density is challenging to measure or estimate on MR imaging, and is variable in individual patients. Breast density may change with surgery or placement of prosthetics, and all of these factors may potentially affect SUV quantification in the evaluation of patients with breast cancer.

STANDARDIZED UPTAKE VALUE: PET-MR IMAGING VERSUS PET-COMPUTED TOMOGRAPHY IN BREAST CANCER

Preliminary work has demonstrated good correlation between SUV measured on PET-MR imaging compared with PET-CT. Most studies compare values by scanning patients first on PET-CT and then on PET-MR imaging. This leads to a time delay between the 2 PET datasets and changes in physiologic concentrations of the radiotracer, which very likely affects the results independent of scanner performance. In 2014, Pace and colleagues[33] reviewed SUV measurements in patients with breast cancer scanned on PET-CT followed by PET-MR imaging an hour later using 2-point Dixon MR imaging sequences that generated a 4 tissue-class attenuation correction map (fat, soft tissue, lungs, air). They found that subjective assessment of lesion localization to anatomic structures was the same between PET-CT and PET-MR imaging. Primary tumors and lymph node uptake was visually scored as having slightly higher contrast on PET-MR imaging. With respect to SUV quantification, the investigators found a significantly higher maximum SUV (SUVmax) for lymph nodes and metastases and no significant change in SUVmax for primary tumors when comparing PET-MR imaging with PET-CT. They found a significantly lower SUV on PET-MR imaging for normal lung, liver, and muscle; no significant difference for spleen; and a higher SUV for left ventricular myocardium. The investigators suggest that these SUV differences likely reflect a combination of time-dependent physiologic and technical scanner factors, and the study design does not allow determination of the impact of the scanner technology alone. They conclude that PET-MR imaging can be used for quantitative analysis in clinical settings but warn that SUV measurements between PET-CT and PET-MR imaging may not be comparable.[33]

In a similar 2015 study by Sawicki and colleagues,[34] 21 subjects with recurrent breast cancer underwent FDG PET-MR imaging immediately following PET-CT. The investigators found a mild but statistically significant increase in SUV on PET-MR imaging for all tumor deposits (SUVmax 5.6 ± 2.8 for PET-MR imaging vs 4.9 ± 1.8 for PET-CT) with strong and significant correlation (r = 0.72, P<.001). Pujara and colleagues[35] studied 35 subjects who underwent FDG PET-CT followed by PET-MR imaging and found statistically significant correlations of SUV measurements for lesions within bone marrow, liver, and lymph nodes (r = 0.74–0.95). They found no statistically significant difference in SUV measurements overall for bone marrow metastases or for lymph node metastases. However, there was a significant difference in average SUVmax for liver metastases (4.96 ± 3.04 for PET-MR imaging vs 7.79 ± 5.78 for PET-CT; P<.05). To what extent this is secondary to segmentation error, tissue attenuation value variability (compared with reality), or time-dependent physiologic differences between PET-CT and PET-MR imaging is uncertain. In contrast to prior studies, PET-MR imaging average SUVmax measurements were slightly lower (eg, 6.25 ± 4.91 for PET-MR imaging vs 6.99 ± 4.63 for PET-CT), as were values (as expected) for normal structures (1.15 ± 1.37 vs 1.60 ± 1.35).

PET-MR IMAGING LESION DETECTION IN BREAST CANCER

A potential advantage of PET-MR imaging compared with PET-CT is in leveraging the MR imaging data to improve lesion detectability. It remains an open question whether or not additional lesion detection with PET-MR imaging will be statistically significant, economically beneficial (in light of the cost of PET-MR imaging), and most importantly advantageous enough to improve patient management decisions and patient outcomes.

In the aforementioned study by Pace and colleagues,[33] lesion detection rates for PET-CT versus PET-MR imaging were reported for 36 subjects undergoing FDG PET-MR imaging following PET-CT. All 74 FDG-avid lesions seen on PET-CT were also visible on PET-MR imaging, including 25 primary tumors, 35 metastatic nodes, and 14 distant metastases. In a study comparing the performance of FDG PET-MR imaging, FDG PET-CT, MR imaging, and CT in the setting of suspected recurrent breast cancer, PET-MR imaging detected 134 lesions, of which 97%, 96%, and 75% were seen on PET-CT, MR imaging, and CT, respectively. The performance of PET-MR imaging and PET-CT for detection of disease recurrence on a per-patient basis is equivalent. On a per-lesion basis, PET-CT was noted to miss 4 bone marrow metastases that were highlighted by the MR imaging portion of PET-MR imaging and found to have some focal FDG uptake that was not initially interpreted as tumor on PET-CT. The investigators note that a limitation of their study was a lack of lung metastases in their subject population, and that small lung lesions can be missed on PET and MR imaging.[34] In a more recent study by Pujara and colleagues[35] that focused on SUV quantification more than analysis of lesions detected, it was noted that during unblinded review, PET-CT initially detected 15 of 16 bone marrow metastases, 6 of 7 liver metastases, and 8 of 8 nonaxillary lymph node metastases that were detected on PET-MR imaging. Therefore, this study further suggests the potential for PET-MR imaging to detect bone marrow and potentially liver metastases that are missed on PET-CT. Finally, Melsaether and colleagues,[36] recently published a formal analysis of 242 distant metastatic lesions, 18 primary breast cancers, and 19 axillary nodes. They found that PET-MR imaging with DWI and contrast-enhanced sequences yielded better sensitivity for liver and possibly bone marrow metastases but potentially worse sensitivity for lung metastases.

Finally, it is worth noting that novel techniques for radiotracer injection may potentially be synergistic, with the added value possibly provided by MR imaging during clinical PET-MR imaging. In 2015, Minamimoto and colleagues[37] reported on a dual-radiotracer technique combining ^{18}F-labeled sodium fluoride (^{18}F-NaF) and FDG injections during PET-CT compared with bone scintigraphy and whole-body MR imaging. The investigators found that combined ^{18}F-NaF-FDG PET-CT offered higher sensitivity for osseous metastasis detection compared with whole-body MR imaging alone but no significant difference compared with a combined read of whole-body MR imaging and bone scintigraphy. In a follow-up abstract published in 2015, the same group published preliminary findings of combined ^{18}F-NaF-FDG PET-MR imaging on a time-of-flight scanner compared with routine bone scintigraphy. Among subjects with osseous metastases, both bone scintigraphy and PET-MR imaging detected lesions. However, more numerous osseous findings were noted on PET-MR imaging in 3 subjects and lesions outside of the skeleton were found on PET-MR imaging in 2 subjects that were not visible on bone scan.[38] A logical follow-up study would be to compare dual-radiotracer PET-MR imaging to PET-CT and bone scintigraphy.

TUMOR STAGING IN BREAST CANCER

There is scant literature directly addressing the possible synergy of PET and MR imaging for T staging of breast cancer. From a technical standpoint, a focused study of the breast is now possible with the advent of PET-MR imaging-compatible breast coils.[39] Although FDG PET is unlikely to improve sensitivity for detection of breast lesions, previously reported improvements in specificity might help to direct biopsies towards areas of more aggressive tumor histology.[40]

ADDITIONAL PET-MR IMAGING APPLICATIONS IN BREAST CANCER: MULTIPARAMETRIC DATASETS

There are few existing data to assess the potential synergistic effects of combining PET and MR imaging quantitative data obtained during a single examination. In a 2014 study by Baba and colleagues,[41] subjects with newly diagnosed breast cancer underwent FDG PET and separate diagnostic breast MR imaging with DWI, and calculation of apparent diffusion coefficient (ADC). A weak inverse correlation between SUV and ADC was reported, and the investigators found that the ratio of SUV to ADC provided very slightly higher accuracy for differentiating between benign and malignant lesions. Unfortunately, this combined parameter did not perform better than SUV or ADC alone in the prediction of overall survival. Miyake and colleagues[42] reported that SUVmax and ADC both change during treatment response before changes in tumor volume are apparent. Finally, Lim and colleagues[43] have demonstrated that a slower decline in SUV, a lesser decline in MR imaging slope on dynamic contrast-enhanced (DCE) MR imaging, and a lower increase in ADC was associated with worse prognosis after the first cycle of neoadjuvant chemotherapy.

Combining these data in a synergistic manner on PET-MR imaging to justify this new technology remains a significant challenge. Future research directions may leverage the ability of PET-MR imaging to acquire kinetic PET data and perform voxelwise correlations between multiparametric datasets with precise image registration and quantitative accuracy. Large-scale multi-institutional studies with advanced data analysis techniques may offer new insights into understanding the significance of the quantitative data that can be obtained from PET-MR imaging. **Figs. 1–3** give examples of PET-MR imaging in patients with breast cancer.

PET-COMPUTED TOMOGRAPHY IN LUNG CANCER

Lung cancer remains the most deadly neoplasm in the United States, affecting both men and women and causing approximately 162,000 deaths in 2015.[1] Lung neoplasms are divided into non-small cell lung cancer (NSCLC) and small cell lung cancer (SCLC). The treatment and prognosis is greatly influenced by tumor type and stage at diagnosis. Evaluation of lung neoplasms has typically been performed using CT to characterize them as malignant, as well as to assess therapeutic response based on lesion change in size on serial imaging. Other imaging characteristics, including shape, edge, cavitation, and location, have not been shown to be as reliable for these purposes.[44,45] Based on lesion size seen on CT alone, 6% to 28% of nodules measuring 5 to 10 mm turn out to be malignant based on subsequent evaluation with invasive procedures or follow-up imaging, with the time interval for follow-up evaluation leading to a delay in the initiation of therapy.[46] The advent of hybrid PET-CT with FDG has an expanding role in this disease given its ability to add functional metabolic information about the tumor to assist in earlier clinical assessment.[47]

FDG PET-CT has been suggested to improve T staging of lung cancer compared with CT alone, particularly for tumors surrounded by atelectasis or abutting the chest wall or mediastinum.[48] FDG PET-CT is both highly sensitive and specific for the diagnosis of pulmonary malignancy.[49–51] However, the sensitivity is lower for small and/or low-attenuation lung cancers, for which morphologic features detected on CT provide an increased role in patient management. The presence or absence of increased radiotracer uptake has the potential to prevent or redirect invasive procedures such as biopsy or resection for histologic sampling. Limitations to the accuracy of FDG PET-CT imaging in lung cancer are similar to other forms of cancer, including false-positive results due to inflammatory or infectious causes and false-negative results within small lesions due to the known lower sensitivity for tumors measuring less than 8 mm.[49] Histologic subtype also influences the uptake of radiotracer, with carcinoid and minimally invasive neoplasms possessing a

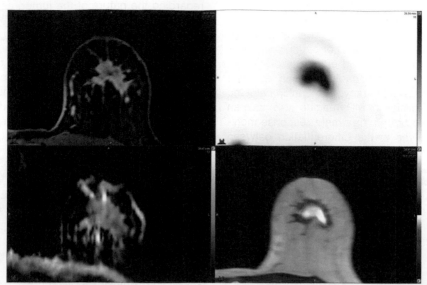

Fig. 1. 54-year-old woman with newly diagnosed left breast cancer. FDG PET-MR imaging performed in the prone position (reoriented) with a dedicated breast coil demonstrates intense FDG uptake in primary tumor on PET and PET-MR images (*top right* and *bottom right*). ADC map MR image (*bottom left*) demonstrates heterogeneous signal intensity with areas of low ADC (*grey-black regions*) within tumor due to high cellularity. Postcontrast T1-weighted MR image (*top left*) demonstrates heterogeneous enhancement within the mass. Prone PET-MR imaging with dedicated breast coil facilitates multiparametric quantitative analysis of primary breast tumors. (*Courtesy of* Dr Amy Melsaether, NYU Langone Medical Center, New York, NY.)

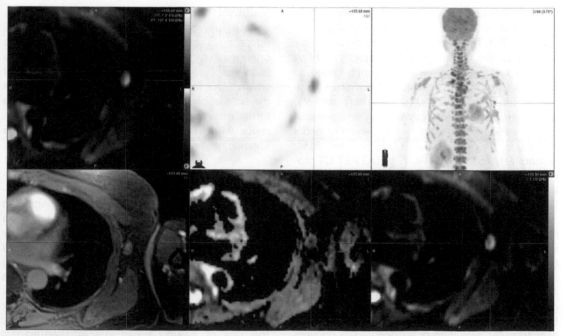

Fig. 2. Left axillary lymph node metastasis in patient presented in **Fig. 1**. FDG PET-MR image (*top left*) and PET images (*top middle* and *top right*) demonstrate intense radiotracer uptake in a borderline prominent left axillary node. T1-weighted fat-suppressed MR image (*bottom left*) demonstrates isointense signal intensity of lymph node relative to skeletal muscle. DWI MR image (*bottom right*) demonstrates high signal intensity of lymph node, and resulting ADC map MR image (*bottom middle*) demonstrates low signal intensity within central portion of the lymph node in keeping with restricted diffusion. (*Courtesy of* Dr Amy Melsaether, NYU Langone Medical Center, New York, NY.)

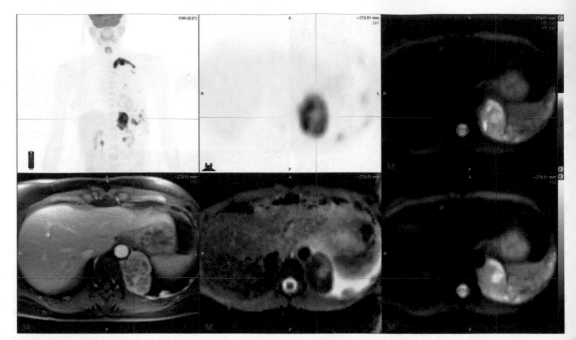

Fig. 3. 51-year-old woman with metastatic left breast cancer. FDG PET images (*top left* and *top middle*) and PET-MR image (*top right*) demonstrate large left lung and left pleural metastases, which demonstrate enhancement on post-contrast T1-weighted fat suppressed MR image (*bottom left*). Note that peripheral rim of FDG uptake in lung metastasis corresponds to regions of high cellularity with restricted diffusion on ADC map MR image (*bottom middle*) derived from DWI MR images (*bottom right*). (*Courtesy of* Dr Amy Melsaether, NYU Langone Medical Center, New York, NY.)

smaller amount of uptake compared with SCLC, leading to lower detection rates on PET-CT.[52–55]

FDG PET-CT has been shown to be useful for diagnosing the spread of lung cancer into hilar, mediastinal, and supraclavicular lymph nodes, in addition to detecting invasion of tumor into the chest wall and mediastinum.[56–59] The sensitivity, specificity, positive predictive value, negative predictive value, and accuracy for detecting nodal spread is 54%, 92%, 74%, 82%, and 81%, respectively, for FDG PET-CT.[60] FDG PET-CT provides additional clinical benefit by guiding selection of the best invasive procedure for lymph node staging.

The incidence of metastasis at the time of diagnosis for lung cancer is high. The most common sites of disease spread are the adrenal glands, bone marrow, liver, and brain. FDG PET-CT has a sensitivity of 100% and a specificity of 80% to 100% for metastatic spread to the adrenal glands.[61,62] For bone marrow metastatic disease, FDG PET has been found to have a similarly high sensitivity for detection of lesions versus conventional bone scintigraphy but with a much higher specificity.[63]

In previously treated patients, the earlier tumor progression can be detected, the faster alternative therapies can be initiated. The potential to monitor treatment response to cytostatic or cytotoxic agents using metabolic markers has many advantages compared to evaluating anatomic changes in tumor size alone. One example of this is in the evaluation of postsurgical patients for which FDG PET-CT can be used to differentiate atelectasis or posttreatment scarring from active tumor recurrence. FDG PET-CT can detect recurrence with a sensitivity of 98% to 100% and a specificity of 62% to 92%.[64,65]

MR IMAGING IN LUNG CANCER

Limitations exist for the use of MR imaging in evaluation of nodules within the lung parenchyma because of the susceptibility artifacts created by air within the lung, low signal-to-nose ratio of aerated lung, and motion artifacts from breathing during image acquisition.[66–69] Several solutions have been proposed to help alleviate these problems, including improved MR imaging hardware, application of novel phased-array receiver coils, the use of newer, faster imaging sequences, including fast spin echo and half-Fourier single-shot turbo spin echo (HASTE) T2-weighted sequences, and DWI.[68–70] The sensitivity of the T2-weighted HASTE MR imaging sequence to detect nodules less than 3 mm, 3 to 5 mm,

5 to 10 mm, and greater than 10 mm has been reported to be 73%, 86%, 96%, and 100%, respectively.[71] In a recent comparison with noncontrast CT and MR imaging using a respiratory-triggered short tau inversion recovery (STIR) MR imaging sequence, there was no difference in the detection of malignant nodules between the 2 sequences, even with the inferior spatial resolution and lower overall nodule detection of MR imaging.[72] DCE MR imaging is another method in development to help differentiate benign versus malignant lung lesions and to evaluate tumor neoangiogenesis.[73,74]

DWI and ADC map images, in which the movement of water molecules within a tissue is measured to determine its cellularity and tissue disorganization, have a sensitivity and specificity of 70% to 89% and 61% to 97%, respectively, in determining the presence of lung neoplasms.[75] The use of dynamic MR imaging techniques has been shown to accurately distinguish malignant from benign lymph nodes with a sensitivity of 94% to 100% and a specificity of 70% to 96%.[75–77]

Due to its improved soft tissue contrast, MR imaging is useful to evaluate tumors in particular areas of the thorax, providing an especially robust modality for diagnostic evaluation. Such tumors include those adjacent to the superior sulcus, where involvement of the chest wall and brachial plexus by tumor can be best appraised by MR imaging, as well as those in the paramediastinal location, in which the relationship with the heart or large vessels is of importance.[78]

PET-MR IMAGING IN LUNG CANCER

Lung cancer is challenging as a diagnostic application for PET-MR imaging due to the known limitations of MR imaging for detection of small and/or low attenuation lung nodules and also due to respiratory motion artifacts that occur in PET and MR imaging. Despite these challenges, potential advantages with respect to chest wall and mediastinal tumor evaluation, combined with the ability of MR imaging to detect brain, bone marrow, adrenal gland, and liver metastases not visible on PET-CT, yields ample room for study of this new modality. Opportunities for gated imaging without additional CT radiation to increase quantitative accuracy of PET and MR imaging data are also potential areas for future research.

STANDARDIZED UPTAKE VALUE: PET-MR IMAGING VERSUS PET- COMPUTED TOMOGRAPHY IN LUNG CANCER

There are currently limited data regarding SUV quantification in lung cancer on PET-MR imaging compared with PET-CT. Given that current clinical PET-MR imaging scanners use a tissue-classification system for estimation of lung density compared with direct measurements obtained on PET-CT, some quantitative differences are expected. In a study focusing on lung nodule detection, Chandarana and colleagues[79] reported that for subjects undergoing PET-MR imaging after PET-CT, SUVmax measurements of lung nodules on PET-MR imaging versus PET-CT were strongly correlated (r = 0.96, $P<.001$) and overall average SUVmax was 16.4 ± 13.6% higher on PET-MR imaging compared with PET-CT. To what extent this difference reflects the more delayed time point of imaging versus differences in attenuation correction factors is not entirely clear. In another study focusing on N staging in which PET-MR imaging was performed after PET-CT, Kohan and colleagues[80] reported that FDG-avid lymph node SUVmax increased from an average of 4.60 on PET-CT up to 5.85 on PET-MR imaging (27.27% higher), with a strong correlation (r = 0.93) again observed. Although most SUV measurements were higher, the investigators point out that misclassification of soft tissue as air in some regions on the MR imaging attenuation map can lead to underestimation of true SUV.

PET-MR IMAGING LESION DETECTION IN LUNG CANCER

Primary tumor detection rates for PET-MR imaging are of interest to clinicians managing patients with lung cancer. It is hypothesized that small lung nodules may be harder to visualize on PET-MR imaging compared with PET-CT based on the known differences between CT and MR imaging. On the other hand, lung cancer has a tendency to spread to the brain, adrenal glands, and bone marrow, which are all areas where MR imaging may potentially perform better. It is, therefore, possible that MR imaging will detect metabolically inactive or minimally active metastases that are missed on PET-CT.

An initial comparison between PET-CT and PET-MR imaging for primary tumor detection noted similar detection rates for primary tumors between the 2 modalities, with identical T staging.[81] With respect to smaller nodules, the performance of PET-MR imaging was worse than PET-CT in a subsequent study by Chandarana and colleagues,[79] for which the sensitivity of PET-MR imaging was 96% for FDG-avid nodules, 70% for all nodules, and 89% for nodules measuring greater than or equal to 5 mm compared with reference standard PET-CT. Only

38% of nodules less than or equal to 4 mm were detected by PET-MR imaging. In a follow-up study at the same institution, Raad and colleagues[82] reported that 97% of nodules missed on PET-MR imaging resolved or remained stable on follow-up, suggestive of benignity. This suggests that most nodules measuring less than 5 mm are either benign or do not contribute significantly to patient management. Further studies are required to explore this issue and to compare the lower sensitivity of PET-MR imaging for small lung nodules against potentially higher sensitivity in other organs such as the brain, liver, adrenal glands, and bone marrow.

With respect to metastatic lymph node detection with PET-MR imaging, preliminary evidence is emerging. In 2014, Heusch and colleagues[83] studied 22 subjects with lung cancer and reported no statistically significant difference between PET-CT and PET-MR imaging for metastatic lymph node detection. PET-MR imaging correctly staged 20 of 22 subjects versus 18 of 22 for PET-CT. The advantage of PET-MR imaging was not only due to the modality. There was time-dependent FDG washout within an inflammatory node in one subject and, in another subject, a lesion was seen on PET-MR imaging that was not visible on PET-CT. Both modalities missed a small supraclavicular lymph node metastasis.

Detection of distant metastases has been studied extensively in the MR imaging literature. Some studies combine PET findings with separately acquired MR imaging, and various MR imaging techniques, including DWI and contrast-enhanced imaging, have been reported. To date, few studies exist for which patients underwent PET-MR imaging in the same imaging session on a single scanner. Preliminary work with integrated PET-MR imaging scanners or software-fused PET and MR imaging datasets has suggested overall equivalence between PET-MR imaging and PET-CT for distant metastasis detection.[83,84] One group has reported that addition of signal intensity quantification on MR imaging may offer higher performance than routine PET-MR imaging or PET-CT.[85] It is likely that large-scale multi-institutional studies will be required to determine if there is a significant true increase in clinically meaningful distant metastasis detection with PET-MR imaging compared with PET-CT.[85]

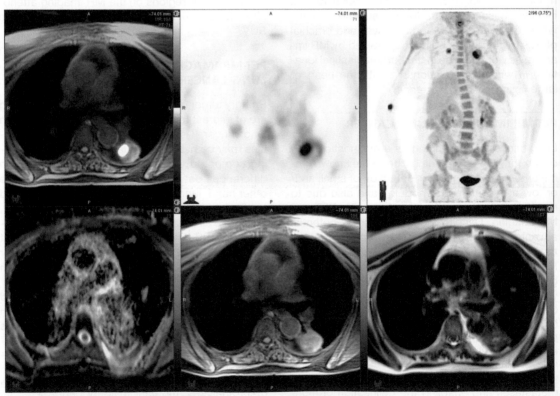

Fig. 4. 78-year-old woman with bilateral lung cancers. FDG PET-MR image (*top left*) and PET images (*top middle* and *top right*) demonstrate peripheral intense radiotracer uptake in left lung tumor that is most intense medially. ADC map MR image (*bottom left*) is degraded by motion artifact, a significant challenge for lung nodule imaging. T1-weighted fat-suppressed MR image (*bottom middle*) and T2-weighted MR image (*bottom right*) demonstrate heterogeneous signal intensity in the left lower lobe mass.

ADDITIONAL PET-MR IMAGING APPLICATIONS IN LUNG CANCER: MULTIPARAMETRIC DATASETS

A potential advantage of PET-MR imaging is that it can deliver quantitatively accurately multiparametric datasets consisting of molecular information from both PET and MR imaging, and that these datasets may improve future patient care. Most of the PET-MR imaging research in this area to date has focused on comparing FDG PET data with that obtained from DWI. The ADC values provided by DWI represent a possible new way to independently or synergistically evaluate tumors during clinical PET-MR imaging.

In 2013, Heusch and colleagues[81] reported a statistically significant inverse correlation between FDG PET SUV and ADC values on PET-MR imaging in subjects with NSCLC. In 2015, Schaarschmidt and colleagues[86] also reported a weak inverse correlation. They suggested the weakness of the correlation suggests that FDG PET and DWI may offer complementary information that may be useful in patients with NSCLC. They discuss that

correlations may vary across histologic subtypes and that further research is required to determine how to use this information. **Figs. 4–6** give examples of PET-MR imaging in patients with lung cancer.

SUMMARY

PET-MR imaging is a promising new modality that brings together the advantages of both MR imaging and PET-CT in a single examination, with few limitations. The potential for increased lesion detection, reduced radiation exposure, improved patient convenience, and improved patient management by leveraging of multiparametric quantitative datasets are all compelling reasons to move forward with clinical PET-MR imaging. That being said, PET-CT is already a highly accurate modality, and large studies will likely be required to demonstrate that PET-MR imaging is worth the additional cost and complexity.

For patients with breast cancer, preliminary research suggests that PET-MR imaging can potentially detect additional tumor deposits in at

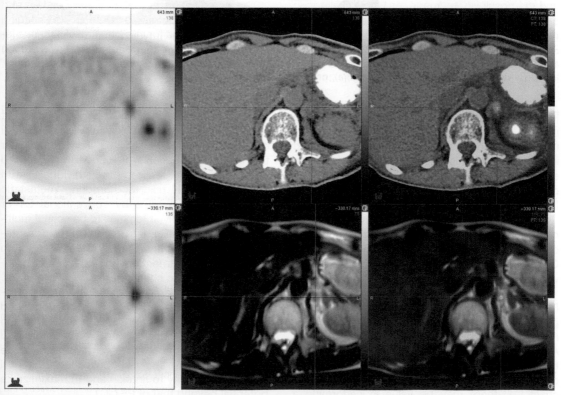

Fig. 5. 64-year-old woman with NSCLC. FDG PET-CT images (*top row*) demonstrate presumed left adrenal gland metastasis, which is not well-delineated on low-dose unenhanced CT image (*top middle*) due to relatively low contrast relative to surrounding diaphragm. FDG PET-MR images (*bottom row*) clearly demonstrate that lesion is a retroperitoneal lymph node (*crosshairs*) just medial to the left adrenal gland (darker inverted V-shaped structure lateral to crosshairs). Improved soft tissue contrast of MR imaging yielded better lesion localization compared with PET-CT.

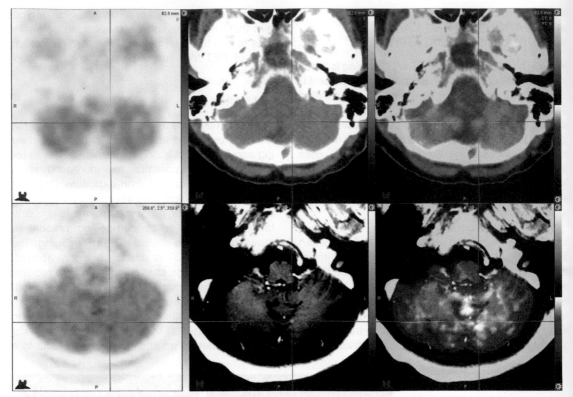

Fig. 6. 70-year-old woman with NSCLC. FDG PET-MR images (*bottom row*) identify an enhancing tiny new left cerebellar brain metastasis seen only on postcontrast T1-weighted MR image (*bottom middle*, see crosshair) and PET-MR image (*bottom right*, see crosshair). Note that the lesion is not visible on PET images (*left column*), low-dose unenhanced CT image (*top middle*), or on PET-CT image (*top right*).

least some patients, particularly in the bone marrow, liver, and brain. A key question is to determine just how often these benefits are realized and in which exact clinical scenarios. It remains to be seen if PET-MR imaging can guide clinicians and patients towards specific therapies or to monitor treatment response in the early stages of therapy. Such applications may require development of new radiotracers that can predict the molecular behavior of breast cancers with higher specificity. Clinical PET-MR imaging in breast cancer is still very much in its infancy.

With respect to lung cancer, it is hard for PET-MR imaging to compete against the near-perfect sensitivity of chest CT for detection of primary lung cancers and metastatic lung nodules. Applications may exist for determining T stage in tumors that abut or invade the mediastinum or chest wall, and in individuals with pre-existing chest CT, there may be value in performing a comprehensive staging study that combines diagnostic MR imaging of the brain, adrenal glands, and liver, with additional bone-marrow specific sequences to comprehensively stage or restage lung cancer. As in the case of breast cancer, it remains

to be seen which exact patient populations and at what particular stages of clinical presentation will benefit from this modality. It is likely that, similar to PET-CT, the benefits of PET-MR imaging will be more likely realized in individuals with moderate-to-high risk for harboring metastatic disease that is invisible by conventional CT or MR imaging. Finally, it remains to be seen if multiparametric PET-MR imaging can be used to predict or monitor treatment responses in an era in which myriad treatment options exist beyond conventional cytotoxic chemotherapy.

Preliminary research has demonstrated a potential added value of PET-MR imaging compared with PET-CT or MR imaging alone in the staging and restaging of patients with breast cancer and lung cancer but much work remains to be done to determine the specific applications that will allow this modality to flourish and to maximize its potential beyond that of PET-CT.

REFERENCES

1. Siegel RL, Miller KD, Jemal A. Cancer statistics, 2015. CA Cancer J Clin 2015;65(1):5–29.

2. Dunphy MPS, Lewis JS. Radiopharmaceuticals in preclinical and clinical development for monitoring of therapy with PET. J Nucl Med 2009;50:106S–21S.

3. Rice SL, Roney CA, Daumar P, et al. The next generation of positron emission tomography radiopharmaceuticals in oncology. Semin Nucl Med 2011;41(4): 265–82.

4. Miller WR, Ellis IO, Sainsbury JR, et al. ABC of breast diseases. Prognostic factors. BMJ 1994;309(6968): 1573–6.

5. Le-Petross CH, Bidaut L, Yang WT. Evolving role of imaging modalities in inflammatory breast cancer. Semin Oncol 2008;35(1):51–63.

6. Yang WT, Le-Petross HT, Macapinlac H, et al. Inflammatory breast cancer: PET/CT, MRI, mammography, and sonography findings. Breast Cancer Res Treat 2008;109(3):417–26.

7. Avril N, Rosé CA, Schelling M, et al. Breast imaging with positron emission tomography and fluorine-18 fluorodeoxyglucose: use and limitations. J Clin Oncol 2000;18(20):3495–502.

8. Heusner TA, Kuemmel S, Umutlu L, et al. Breast cancer staging in a single session: whole-body PET/CT mammography. J Nucl Med 2008;49(8):1215–22.

9. Scheidhauer K, Walter C, Seemann MD. FDG PET and other imaging modalities in the primary diagnosis of suspicious breast lesions. Eur J Nucl Med Mol Imaging 2004;31(Suppl 1):S70–9.

10. Uematsu T, Kasami M, Yuen S. Comparison of FDG PET and MRI for evaluating the tumor extent of breast cancer and the impact of FDG PET on the systemic staging and prognosis of patients who are candidates for breast-conserving therapy. Breast Cancer 2009;16(2):97–104.

11. Heusner TA, Freudenberg LS, Kuehl H, et al. Whole-body PET/CT-mammography for staging breast cancer: initial results. Br J Radiol 2008;81(969):743–8.

12. Torizuka T, Zasadny KR, Recker B, et al. Untreated primary lung and breast cancers: correlation between F-18 FDG kinetic rate constants and findings of in vitro studies. Radiology 1998;207(3):767–74.

13. Kumar R, Loving VA, Chauhan A, et al. Potential of dual-time-point imaging to improve breast cancer diagnosis with (18)F-FDG PET. J Nucl Med 2005; 46(11):1819–24.

14. Mavi A, Urhan M, Yu JQ, et al. Dual time point 18F-FDG PET imaging detects breast cancer with high sensitivity and correlates well with histologic subtypes. J Nucl Med 2006;47(9):1440–6.

15. Wahl RL, Siegel BA, Coleman RE, et al. Prospective multicenter study of axillary nodal staging by positron emission tomography in breast cancer: a report of the staging breast cancer with PET Study Group. J Clin Oncol 2004;22(2):277–85.

16. Schwarz-Dose J, Untch M, Tiling R, et al. Monitoring primary systemic therapy of large and locally advanced breast cancer by using sequential positron emission tomography imaging with [18F]fluorodeoxyglucose. J Clin Oncol 2009;27(4):535–41.

17. Rousseau C, Devillers A, Sagan C, et al. Monitoring of early response to neoadjuvant chemotherapy in stage II and III breast cancer by [18F]fluorodeoxyglucose positron emission tomography. J Clin Oncol 2006;24(34):5366–72.

18. Kamel EM, Wyss MT, Fehr MK, et al. [18F]-Fluorodeoxyglucose positron emission tomography in patients with suspected recurrence of breast cancer. J Cancer Res Clin Oncol 2003;129(3):147–53.

19. Eubank WB, Mankoff D, Bhattacharya M, et al. Impact of FDG PET on defining the extent of disease and on the treatment of patients with recurrent or metastatic breast cancer. AJR Am J Roentgenol 2004;183(2):479–86.

20. Tateishi U, Gamez C, Dawood S, et al. Bone metastases in patients with metastatic breast cancer: morphologic and metabolic monitoring of response to systemic therapy with integrated PET/CT. Radiology 2008;247(1):189–96.

21. Siggelkow W, Zimny M, Faridi A, et al. The value of positron emission tomography in the follow-up for breast cancer. Anticancer Res 2003;23(2C): 1859–67.

22. Du Y, Cullum I, Illidge TM, et al. Fusion of metabolic function and morphology: sequential [18F]fluorodeoxyglucose positron-emission tomography/computed tomography studies yield new insights into the natural history of bone metastases in breast cancer. J Clin Oncol 2007;25(23):3440–7.

23. Tillman GF, Orel SG, Schnall MD, et al. Effect of breast magnetic resonance imaging on the clinical management of women with early-stage breast carcinoma. J Clin Oncol 2002;20(16):3413–23.

24. Lehman CD, DeMartini W, Anderson BO, et al. Indications for breast MRI in the patient with newly diagnosed breast cancer. J Natl Compr Canc Netw 2009;7(2):193–201.

25. Weinstein S, Rosen M. Breast MR imaging: current indications and advanced imaging techniques. Radiol Clin North Am 2010;48(5):1013–42.

26. Zeppa R. Vascular response of breast to estrogen. J Clin Endocrinol Metab 1969;29(5):695–700.

27. Vogel PM, Georgiade NG, Fetter BF, et al. The correlation of histologic-changes in the human-breast with the menstrual-cycle. Am J Pathol 1981;104(1): 23–34.

28. Giess CS, Yeh ED, Raza S, et al. Background parenchymal enhancement at breast MR imaging: normal patterns, diagnostic challenges, and potential for false-positive and false-negative interpretation. Radiographics 2014;34(1):234–47.

29. Vag T, Baltzer PA, Dietzel M, et al. Kinetic characteristics of ductal carcinoma in situ (DCIS) in dynamic breast MRI using computer-assisted analysis. Acta Radiol 2010;51(9):955–61.

30. Kvistad KA, Rydland J, Vainio J, et al. Breast lesions: evaluation with dynamic contrast-enhanced T1-weighted MR imaging and with T2*-weighted first-pass perfusion MR imaging. Radiology 2000; 216(2):545–53.

31. Kim JA, Son EJ, Youk JH, et al. MRI findings of pure ductal carcinoma in situ: kinetic characteristics compared according to lesion type and histopathologic factors. AJR Am J Roentgenol 2011;196(6): 1450–6.

32. Kvistad KA, Rydland J, Smethurst HB, et al. Axillary lymph node metastases in breast cancer: preoperative detection with dynamic contrast-enhanced MRI. Eur Radiol 2000;10(9):1464–71.

33. Pace L, Nicolai E, Luongo A, et al. Comparison of whole-body PET/CT and PET/MRI in breast cancer patients: lesion detection and quantitation of 18F-deoxyglucose uptake in lesions and in normal organ tissues. Eur J Radiol 2014;83(2):289–96.

34. Sawicki LM, Grueneisen J, Schaarschmidt BM, et al. Evaluation of (18)F-FDG PET/MRI, (18)F-FDG PET/CT, MRI, and CT in whole-body staging of recurrent breast cancer. Eur J Radiol 2016;85(2):459–65.

35. Pujara AC, Raad RA, Ponzo F, et al. Standardized uptake values from PET/MRI in metastatic breast cancer: an organ-based comparison with PET/CT. Breast J 2016;22(3):264–73.

36. Melsaether AN, Raad RA, Pujara AC, et al. Comparison of whole-body F FDG PET/MR imaging and whole-body F FDG PET/CT in terms of lesion detection and radiation dose in patients with breast cancer. Radiology 2016;151155. [Epub ahead of print].

37. Minamimoto R, Mosci C, Jamali M, et al. Semiquantitative analysis of the biodistribution of the combined (1)(8)F-NaF and (1)(8)F-FDG administration for PET/CT imaging. J Nucl Med 2015;56(5): 688–94.

38. Iagaru A, Minamimoto R, Levin C, et al. The potential of TOF PET-MRI for reducing artifacts in PET images. EJNMMI Phys 2015;2(Suppl 1):A77.

39. Dregely I, Lanz T, Metz S, et al. A 16-channel MR coil for simultaneous PET/MR imaging in breast cancer. Eur Radiol 2015;25(4):1154–61.

40. Moy L, Noz ME, Maguire GQ Jr, et al. Role of fusion of prone FDG-PET and magnetic resonance imaging of the breasts in the evaluation of breast cancer. Breast J 2010;16(4):369–76.

41. Baba S, Isoda T, Maruoka Y, et al. Diagnostic and prognostic value of pretreatment SUV in 18F-FDG/ PET in breast cancer: comparison with apparent diffusion coefficient from diffusion-weighted MR imaging. J Nucl Med 2014;55(5):736–42.

42. Miyake KK, Nakamoto Y, Kanao S, et al. Journal club: diagnostic value of (18)F-FDG PET/CT and MRI in predicting the clinicopathologic subtypes of invasive breast cancer. AJR Am J Roentgenol 2014;203(2):272–9.

43. Lim I, Noh WC, Park J, et al. The combination of FDG PET and dynamic contrast-enhanced MRI improves the prediction of disease-free survival in patients with advanced breast cancer after the first cycle of neoadjuvant chemotherapy. Eur J Nucl Med Mol Imaging 2014;41(10):1852–60.

44. Brandman S, Ko JP. Pulmonary nodule detection, characterization, and management with multidetector computed tomography. J Thorac Imaging 2011; 26(2):90–105.

45. Zhao F, Yan SX, Wang GF, et al. CT features of focal organizing pneumonia: an analysis of consecutive histopathologically confirmed 45 cases. Eur J Radiol 2014;83(1):73–8.

46. Zhang ZW, Rong EG, Shi MX, et al. Expression and functional analysis of Kruppel-like factor 2 in chicken adipose tissue. J Anim Sci 2014;92(11): 4797–805.

47. Eubank WB, Mankoff DA, Schmiedl UP, et al. Imaging of oncologic patients: benefit of combined CT and FDG PET in the diagnosis of malignancy. Am J Roentgenol 1998;171(4):1103–10.

48. De Wever W, Ceyssens S, Mortelmans L, et al. Additional value of PET-CT in the staging of lung cancer: comparison with CT alone, PET alone and visual correlation of PET and CT. Eur Radiol 2007;17(1):23–32.

49. Gould MK, Maclean CC, Kuschner WG, et al. Accuracy of positron emission tomography for diagnosis of pulmonary nodules and mass lesions: a meta-analysis. JAMA 2001;285(7):914–24.

50. Lowe VJ, Fletcher JW, Gobar L, et al. Prospective investigation of positron emission tomography in lung nodules. J Clin Oncol 1998;16(3):1075–84.

51. Patz EF, Lowe VJ, Hoffman JM, et al. Focal pulmonary abnormalities: evaluation with F-18 fluorodeoxyglucose PET scanning. Radiology 1993;188(2): 487–90.

52. Erasmus JJ, McAdams HP, Patz EF Jr, et al. Evaluation of primary pulmonary carcinoid tumors using FDG PET. Am J Roentgenol 1998;170(5):1369–73.

53. Higashi K, Ueda Y, Seki H, et al. Fluorine-18-FDG PET imaging is negative in bronchioloalveolar lung carcinoma. J Nucl Med 1998;39(6):1016–20.

54. Kim BT, Kim Y, Lee KS, et al. Localized form of bronchioloalveolar carcinoma: FDG PET findings. Am J Roentgenol 1998;170(4):935–9.

55. Henschke CI, Yankelevitz DF, Kostis WJ. CT screening for lung cancer. Semin Ultrasound CT MR 2003;24(1):23–32.

56. Antoch G, Stattaus J, Nemat AT, et al. Non-small cell lung cancer: dual-modality PET/CT in preoperative staging. Radiology 2003;229(2):526–33.

57. Birim O, Kappetein AP, Stijnen T, et al. Meta-analysis of positron emission tomographic and computed tomographic imaging in detecting mediastinal lymph node metastases in nonsmall cell lung cancer. Ann Thorac Surg 2005;79(1):375–82.

58. Halter G, Buck AK, Schirrmeister H, et al. Lymph node staging in lung cancer using [F-18]FDG-PET. Thorac Cardiovasc Surg 2004;52(2):96–101.

59. Lardinois D, Weder W, Hany TF, et al. Staging of non-small-cell lung cancer with integrated positron-emission tomography and computed tomography. N Engl J Med 2003;348(25):2500–7.

60. Bille A, Pelosi E, Skanjeti A, et al. Preoperative intra-thoracic lymph node staging in patients with non-small-cell lung cancer: accuracy of integrated positron emission tomography and computed to-mography. Eur J Cardiothorac Surg 2009;36(3): 440–5.

61. Erasmus JJ, Patz EF Jr, McAdams HP, et al. Evalua-tion of adrenal masses in patients with bronchogenic carcinoma using F-18-fluorodeoxy-glucose positron emission tomography. Am J Roentgenol 1997; 168(5):1357–60.

62. Marom EM, McAdams HP, Erasmus JJ, et al. Stag-ing non-small cell lung cancer with whole-body PET. Radiology 1999;212(3):803–9.

63. Bury T, Corhay JL, Duysinx B, et al. Value of FDG-PET in detecting residual or recurrent nonsmall cell lung cancer. Eur Respir J 1999;14(6):1376–80.

64. Hellwig D, Gröschel A, Graeter TP, et al. Diagnostic performance and prognostic impact of FDG-PET in suspected recurrence of surgically treated non-small cell lung cancer. Eur J Nucl Med Mol Imaging 2006;33(1):13–21.

65. Ryu JS, Choi NC, Fischman AJ, et al. FDG-PET in staging and restaging non-small cell lung cancer af-ter neoadjuvant chemoradiotherapy: correlation with histopathology. Lung Cancer 2002;35(2):179–87.

66. Bergin CJ, Glover GH, Pauly JM. Lung parenchyma: magnetic-susceptibility in MR imaging. Radiology 1991;180(3):845–8.

67. Lauenstein TC, Goehde SC, Herborn CU, et al. Whole-body MR imaging: evaluation of patients for metastases. Radiology 2004;233(1):139–48.

68. Ohno Y, Oshio K, Uematsu H, et al. Single-shot half-Fourier RARE sequence with ultra-short inter-echo spacing for lung imaging. J Magn Reson Imaging 2004;20(2):336–9.

69. Attenberger U, Catana C, Chandarana H, et al. Whole-body FDG PET-MR oncologic imaging: pit-falls in clinical interpretation related to inaccurate MR-based attenuation correction. Abdom Imaging 2015;40(6):1374–86.

70. Kurihara Y, Matsuoka S, Yamashiro T, et al. MRI of pulmonary nodules. Am J Roentgenol 2014;202(3): W210–6.

71. Schroeder T, Ruehm SG, Debatin JF, et al. Detection of pulmonary nodules using a 2D HASTE MR sequence: comparison with MDCT. Am J Roent-genol 2005;185(4):979–84.

72. Koyama H, Ohno Y, Kono A, et al. Quantitative and qualitative assessment of non-contrast-enhanced pulmonary MR imaging for management of pulmo-nary nodules in 161 subjects. Eur Radiol 2008; 18(10):2120–31.

73. Fujimoto K, Abe T, Müller NL, et al. Small peripheral pulmonary carcinomas evaluated with dynamic MR imaging: correlation with tumor vascularity and prognosis. Radiology 2003;227(3):786–93.

74. Kono R, Fujimoto K, Terasaki H, et al. Dynamic MRI of solitary pulmonary nodules: comparison of enhancement patterns of malignant and benign small peripheral lung lesions. Am J Roentgenol 2007;188(1):26–36.

75. Uto T, Takehara Y, Nakamura Y, et al. Higher sensi-tivity and specificity for diffusion-weighted imaging of malignant lung lesions without apparent diffusion coefficient quantification. Radiology 2009;252(1): 247–54.

76. Koyama H, Ohno Y, Aoyama N, et al. Comparison of STIR turbo SE imaging and diffusion-weighted imag-ing of the lung: capability for detection and subtype classification of pulmonary adenocarcinomas. Eur Radiol 2010;20(4):790–800.

77. Mori T, Nomori H, Ikeda K, et al. Diffusion-weighted magnetic resonance imaging for diagnosing malig-nant pulmonary nodules/masses: comparison with positron emission tomography. J Thorac Oncol 2008;3(4):358–64.

78. Schrevens L, Lorent N, Dooms C, et al. The role of PET scan in diagnosis, staging, and management of non-small cell lung cancer. Oncologist 2004; 9(6):633–43.

79. Chandarana H, Heacock L, Rakheja R, et al. Pulmo-nary nodules in patients with primary malignancy: comparison of hybrid PET/MR and PET/CT imaging. Radiology 2013;268(3):874–81.

80. Kohan AA, Kolthammer JA, Vercher-Conejero JL, et al. N staging of lung cancer patients with PET/MRI using a three-segment model attenuation correction algorithm: initial experience. Eur Radiol 2013;23(11):3161–9.

81. Heusch P, Köhler J, Wittsack HJ, et al. Hybrid [(1)(8) F]-FDG PET/MRI including non-Gaussian diffusion-weighted imaging (DWI): preliminary results in non-small cell lung cancer (NSCLC). Eur J Radiol 2013; 82(11):2055–60.

82. Raad RA, Friedman KP, Heacock L, et al. Outcome of small lung nodules missed on hybrid PET/MRI in patients with primary malignancy. J Magn Reson Im-aging 2016;43(2):504–11.

83. Heusch P, Buchbender C, Köhler J, et al. Thoracic staging in lung cancer: prospective comparison of 18F-FDG PET/MR imaging and 18F-FDG PET/CT. J Nucl Med 2014;55(3):373–8.

84. Lee SM, Goo JM, Park CM, et al. Preoperative stag-ing of non-small cell lung cancer: prospective com-parison of PET/MR and PET/CT. Eur Radiol 2016. [Epub ahead of print].

85. Ohno Y, Koyama H, Yoshikawa T, et al. Three-way comparison of whole-body MR, coregistered whole-body FDG PET/MR, and integrated whole-body FDG PET/CT Imaging: TNM and stage assessment capability for non-small cell lung cancer patients. Radiology 2015;275(3):849–61.

86. Schaarschmidt BM, Buchbender C, Nensa F, et al. Correlation of the apparent diffusion coefficient (ADC) with the standardized uptake value (SUV) in lymph node metastases of non-small cell lung cancer (NSCLC) patients using hybrid 18F-FDG PET/MRI. PLoS One 2015;10(1):e0116277.

PET/MR Imaging in Cancers of the Gastrointestinal Tract

Raj Mohan Paspulati, MD, FSAR[a],*, Amit Gupta, MD[b]

KEYWORDS

- PET/MR imaging • Gastrointestinal tract malignancy • [18F]-2-fluoro-2-deoxy-d-glucose PET
- Rectal carcinoma • Liver tumors • Treatment response

KEY POINTS

- PET/MR imaging is an evolving hybrid imaging technique with potential use in initial staging and follow-up of gastrointestinal tract malignancies.
- High soft tissue contrast resolution of MR imaging is an advantage over computed tomography for T staging of rectal carcinoma and characterization of liver lesions.
- Functional MR imaging techniques such as diffusion-weighted imaging adds to metabolic information from [18F]-2-fluoro-2-deoxy-D-glucose PET in more accurate assessment of tumor response and local recurrence after treatment of colorectal carcinoma.
- Approval of new radiotracers will widen the scope of PET/MR imaging application in non–[18F]-2-fluoro-2-deoxy-D-glucose–avid tumors.

INTRODUCTION

PET/MR imaging is an emerging new technology that combines the anatomic and functional capabilities of MR imaging and the metabolic information of PET into a single examination. This new hybrid modality was recently introduced into the clinical arena, and since then clinical data regarding the feasibility and potential applications of PET/MR imaging have been rapidly emerging, especially in oncology.[1–3] Over the last 2 decades, [18F]-2-fluoro-2-deoxy-D-glucose (FDG) PET/CT, a combination of PET using a glucose analogue FDG and CT, has established itself as a powerful tool in staging, restaging, treatment planning, and monitoring response in many malignancies.[4,5] However, the anatomic information provided by the low-dose, noncontrast CT component of the PET/CT examination is often insufficient to

determine the extent of local tumor invasion or to characterize incidental lesions. In contrast, MR imaging with its superior soft-tissue contrast resolution, multiplanar imaging acquisition capability, and functional imaging capability allows better anatomic visualization of soft tissue and musculoskeletal structures compared with CT.[6,7] Moreover, MR imaging is devoid of ionizing radiation of CT; therefore, PET/MR imaging has potential of reducing radiation exposure to vulnerable pediatric and pregnant oncology populations, which often require frequent follow-up studies.[8] Therefore, PET/MR imaging integrates the advantages of MR imaging and PET and has great potential in improving lesion detection and diagnostic performance. Regardless of these advantages, PET/MR imaging is still in its nascent stage, and further prospective studies are required

The authors have nothing to disclose.
[a] Division of Abdominal Imaging, Department of Radiology, University Hospitals Case Western Reserve University, 11100 Euclid Avenue, Cleveland, OH 44106, USA; [b] Department of Radiology, University Hospitals Case Western Reserve University, 11100 Euclid Avenue, Cleveland, OH 44106, USA
* Corresponding author.
E-mail address: Raj.Paspulati@UHhospitals.org

PET Clin 11 (2016) 403–423
http://dx.doi.org/10.1016/j.cpet.2016.05.004

to fully establish its potential value compared with PET/CT. In this article, the current literature and potential clinical applications of PET/MR imaging in common malignancies involving the gastrointestinal (GI) tract, including liver, biliary tract, pancreatic, and colorectal tumors, are discussed.

TECHNICAL BACKGROUND
PET/MR Imaging Systems

There are 2 commercially available PET/MR imaging scanners classified as sequential and simultaneous systems.[9] The sequential PET/MR imaging has separate PET and MR imaging elements physically separated by a rotating table. The sequential design has a relatively simple construction and only minor modifications to the preexisting hardware and software but is more prone to image misregistration because of the temporal separation of the PET and MR imaging data. This design also requires a much larger area to accommodate both scanners.[10–12]

The simultaneous or integrated PET/MR imaging scanner has a complex structure with PET detectors inserted between the gradient and radiofrequency body coils of the MR imaging scanner. There is need for modifications to avoid electromagnetic interactions between 2 components and use of magnetic field–insensitive avalanche photodiodes and silicon photomultiplier detectors, which are immune to magnetic field effects. The simultaneous data acquisition has the advantages of shorter scan times and reduced misregistration as well as alleviation of the need for a large room. However, respiratory motion artifacts still remain a problem, particularly in the upper abdomen.[13–15]

PET/MR IMAGING PROTOCOL

Integrated whole-body PET/MR imaging typically consists of 2 parts, whole-body PET/MR imaging and dedicated regional MR imaging. Generally, the whole body portion of the examination is more or less the same for most malignancies, but the region-specific sequences vary with location of tumor and the clinical indication for the examination, which can potentially increase the duration of the examination. The future success of PET/MR imaging depends on workflow efficiency; therefore, a typical whole-body scan should not exceed 20 to 30 minutes.[16,17] Additionally, the length of dedicated MR imaging may be reduced by tailoring the regional MR imaging sequences according to the clinical indication. A lengthy study may not be well tolerated by some oncologic patients.[18]

Whole-Body PET/MR Imaging Protocol

Optional whole-body MR imaging sequences include DWI and short tau inversion recovery (STIR) imaging.

Whole-body DWI, which may improve diagnostic accuracy in tumors such as lymphoma,[19,20] and whole-body coronal STIR imaging have been found to improve detection of osseous lesions.[21]

Region-Specific Dedicated MR Imaging Protocols

Dedicated MR imaging sequences of regions of interest are required to better assess the local extent of disease and T staging (**Boxes 1** and **2**). DWI with apparent diffusion coefficient (ADC) maps is routinely performed, as it is useful to assess the cellularity of the primary tumor and to distinguish posttreatment inflammation and fibrosis from viable neoplasm.[22–24] DWI also improves the sensitivity of detection for lymph node and peritoneal metastases.[25,26]

Workflow

The imaging time of PET/MR imaging dependents the number of MR imaging sequences and the duration of each MR imaging sequence (**Figs. 1** and **2**). The examination protocol should be tailored to answer the specific clinical question for that particular patient.

Box 1
Protocol for GI malignancy (liver, biliary tract, and pancreatic) abdominal MR imaging

- Axial and coronal heavily T2-weighted images without fat suppression.

- Axial T1-weighted in and out of phase chemical shift gradient recalled echo (GRE) images.

- Axial DWI (b values of 50, 600, and 800).

- Axial 3-dimensional T1-weighted GRE images with fat suppression before contrast administration.

- Axial 3-dimensional T1-weighted GRE images with fat suppression acquired dynamically during multiple phases after intravenous administration of a gadolinium-based contrast agent.

- Axial 3-dimensional T1-weighted GRE images with fat suppression acquired during the hepatobiliary phase at 15 to 20 minutes if a hepatobiliary-specific gadolinium-based contrast agent was administered.

- MRCP is optional and not routinely performed.

Box 2
Protocol for rectal carcinoma pelvic MR imaging

- Axial, coronal, and sagittal heavily T2-weighted images without fat suppression.
- Axial and sagittal high-resolution T2-weighted fast spin echo images without fat saturation.
- Axial DWI (b values of 50, 600, and 1000).
- Axial 3-dimensional T1-weighted GRE images with fat suppression before contrast administration.
- Axial 3-dimensional T1-weighted GRE images with fat suppression acquired dynamically during multiple phases after intravenous administration of a gadolinium-based contrast agent.
- Sagittal and coronal-delayed phase postcontrast T1-weighted GRE images.
- Coronal STIR images of whole body to assess osseous structures.

CLINICAL APPLICATIONS

Accurate diagnosis, staging, response assessment, and restaging form the basis for the optimal treatment of cancer patients and determine the therapeutic approach. Cross-sectional imaging coupled with the metabolic information of PET play a crucial role in cancer staging. The TNM staging system is one globally recognized standard for classifying the extent of spread of cancer. PET/CT has already been accepted as a robust tool in oncology, outperforming conventional imaging modalities. It too has limitations because of poor soft tissue resolution of CT, lack of specificity of FDG uptake, and variable FDG avidity of some cancers. These limitations can be countered by substituting CT with MR imaging, which can be particularly useful in hepatic and rectal malignancies.

LIVER
Hepatocellular Carcinoma

Hepatocellular carcinoma (HCC) is the sixth most common malignancy and a leading cause of mortality in patients with cirrhosis.[27]

Currently, contrast-enhanced MR imaging, and, to a lesser extent, triple-phase contrast-enhanced CT, remain the mainstay for detection of HCC. A definitive diagnosis of HCC can be made in lesions measuring greater than 1 cm without a tissue diagnosis by demonstrating arterial phase hyperenhancement and venous or delayed phase washout.[28–30] Use of functional imaging techniques such as DWI and hepatobiliary contrast agents such as gadolinium-ethoxybenzyl-diethylenetriamine pentaacetic acid or gadobenate acid can further improve the diagnosis of indeterminate hepatic lesions.[31–33] MR imaging is also significantly better than CT in lesion characterization. A study performed by Holalkere and colleagues[34] found sensitivity, specificity, positive predictive value, and negative predictive value in differentiating benign from malignant lesions of 83.3%, 97.5%, 92.1%, and 94.4%, respectively, for MR imaging compared with 81.2%, 77.3%, 60.5%, and 90.6%, respectively, for multidetector CT.

The role of PET/MR imaging in initial diagnosis of HCC of the liver has yet to be established. FDG PET has limited utility in diagnosing HCC because of its low sensitivity. This low sensitivity is caused by preferential FDG uptake in poorly differentiated and histopathologic high-grade HCC (**Fig. 3**) and no uptake in well-differentiated and low-grade HCC[35] (**Fig. 4**). The tumor size is also a key factor, as FDG has low sensitivity and high false-negative uptake in HCC less than 5 cm.[36] Non-FDG radiotracers such as [11C]-acetate and [18F]-choline are reported to have high sensitivity for low-grade HCC, as uptake of these radiotracers is related to de novo lipid synthesis. The radiotracer

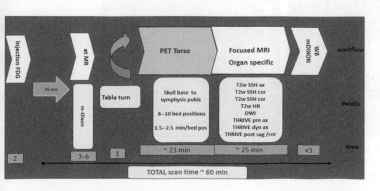

Fig. 1. Sequential type PET/MR imaging workflow. This includes whole-body (WB) and organ-specific MR imaging. atMR, attenuation correction MR; DWI, diffusion weighted imaging; T2 SSH, T2 single shot; THRIVE, T1W high resolution isotropic volume examination; WB m DIXON, whole body m Dixon.

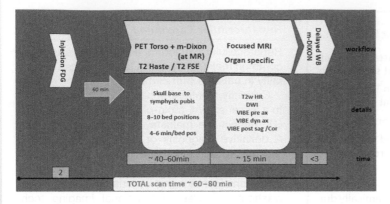

Fig. 2. Simultaneous type PET/MR imaging workflow. This includes whole-body (WB) and organ specific MR imaging. DWI, diffusion weighted imaging; T2 FSE, T2 fast spin echo; T2 Haste, T2 half fourier acquisition single shot turbo spin echo; VIBE, volumetric interpolated breath hold examination; WB m DIXON, whole body m Dixon.

[11C]-acetate has the disadvantage of a short half-life of 20 minutes and need for an on-site cyclotron. Similar to FDG, these radiotracers also have a low sensitivity for small HCC measuring less than 2 cm.[37,38]

Imaging also plays an important role in assessment of treatment response of primary tumor to locoregional treatment and to systemic chemotherapy. Evaluation of response to various types of locoregional therapy of HCC by contrast-enhanced CT or MR imaging alone is limited, as alterations in tumor size and enhancement are less reliable because of posttreatment changes. Use of FDG PET in addition to MR imaging would be beneficial for better assessment of tumor response (Fig. 5).[39,40] Despite the limitation of FDG PET in detection of primary HCC, it has been a valuable tool in detection of extrahepatic metastases before liver transplantation and in posttransplant patients.[41] This discrepancy occurs because extrahepatic disease is more frequently associated with high-grade and large size primary HCC.[42] Lymph nodes are the second most common site of metastatic disease in HCC (after the lung), and nodal involvement is associated with lower survival rates. Lymph node involvement is usually seen with larger tumor size (>5 cm), presence of microvascular invasion, and poorly differentiated histology.[43–45] Differentiation of reactive from metastatic lymph

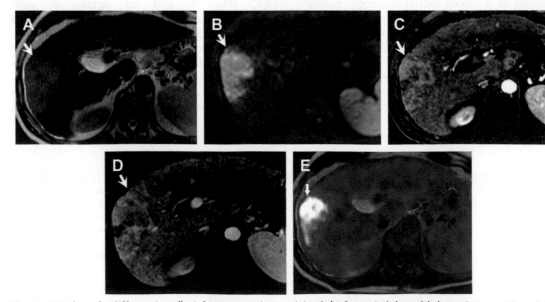

Fig. 3. HCC (poorly differentiated). A large mass (arrows) in right hepatic lobe with hyperintense T2-weighted signal intensity relative to liver (A), restricted diffusion (B), arterial phase enhancement (C), and heterogeneous venous phase washout (D) on MR imaging shows intense FDG uptake on fused PET/MR image (E).

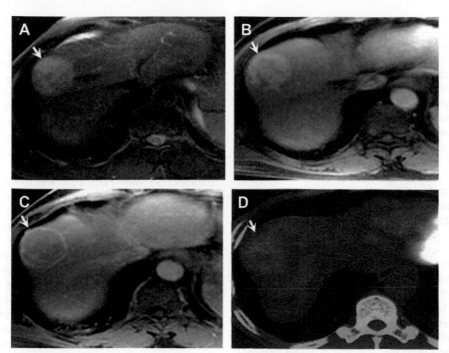

Fig. 4. HCC (well-differentiated). A well-defined mass (*arrows*) in right hepatic lobe with hyperintense T2-weighted signal intensity relative to liver (*A*), intense arterial phase enhancement (*B*), and delayed phase washout with enhancing pseudocapsule formation (*C*) on MR imaging shows no significant FDG uptake on PET/CT image (*D*).

nodes by size criteria is suboptimal, and use of FDG PET in addition to functional MR imaging sequences such as DWI improves the sensitivity of detection of lymph node metastases.[42,46,47] FDG PET is also reported to be of value in predicting treatment response to locoregional treatment and overall survival rates. Several studies have shown that HCC with a low tumor-to-normal liver standardized uptake value ratio had better response to locoregional treatment such as transarterial chemoembolization.[48]

In light of the above discussion, it can be inferred that MR imaging in conjunction with FDG PET has a potential role in selected patients in differentiating high- and low-grade tumors and in improved detection of extrahepatic metastases in both pre–liver transplant patients and during follow-up for posttransplant extrahepatic tumor recurrence. PET/MR imaging can be a single substitute examination to separate PET/CT and MR imaging examinations for initial staging, particularly when disseminated disease is suspected.

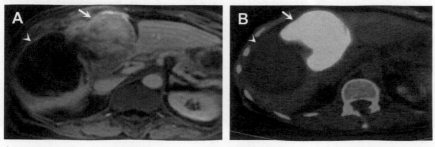

Fig. 5. Partial response of a large poorly differentiated HCC to transarterial chemoembolization. Contrast-enhanced T1-weighted MR image (*A*) shows no enhancement in treated the right half of the lesion (*arrowhead*) and persistent enhancement in other viable half of the lesion (*arrow*). Corresponding PET/CT image (*B*) shows no FDG uptake in nonenhancing region (*arrowhead*) of lesion and intense FDG uptake in enhancing half of lesion (*arrow*).

Liver Metastases

Liver is the most common site for metastases from GI tract malignancies, with nearly more than 50% of colorectal carcinoma patients having hepatic metastases either synchronously or metachronously.[49] Liver is also a common site for metastases in leading extra-abdominal primary malignancies such as breast and lung carcinomas. Improved survival rates in metastatic colorectal carcinoma are caused by new chemotherapeutic regimens and more aggressive surgical approaches to hepatic metastases.[50] Imaging plays an important role in the workup of these patients in initial staging and during follow-up to assess treatment response and recurrent metastatic disease.

Contrast-enhanced CT is the primary imaging modality for initial staging of GI tract malignancy and detection, localization, and characterization of liver lesions. Indeterminate liver lesions on contrast-enhanced CT are further characterized by either MR imaging or FDG PET. Several studies compared the efficacy of these different imaging modalities in detection of liver metastases. FDG PET/CT is found to be superior to contrast-enhanced CT but less sensitive than contrast-enhanced MR imaging in detection of small hepatic metastases measuring less than 1 cm.[51] This is especially found to be the case

with contrast-enhanced MR imaging using liver-specific contrast agents. Detection of these small metastases has an impact on the type of treatment modality. Hybrid PET/MR imaging has the advantages of both MR imaging and FDG PET in not only detection of metastases but also in characterization of non–FDG-avid lesions.[52,53] Beiderwellen et al[43] showed higher sensitivity and accuracy of hybrid PET/MR imaging than PET/CT in detection of liver metastases. Use of liver-specific contrast-enhanced MR imaging in conjunction with FDG PET will further improve the efficacy in detection of liver metastases and follow-up after locoregional treatment of hepatic metastases (**Figs. 6–8**). Several studies found increased sensitivity and negative predictive value of MR imaging with hepatobiliary contrast agents in detection of small liver metastases measuring less than 1 cm compared with PET/CT.[44] Hybrid PET/MR imaging with hepatobiliary contrast agents has a potential advantage over PET/CT and MR imaging in detection of small metastases.[45] FDG PET/CT also has a high percentage of false-negative results with mucinous and hypocellular liver metastases.[54,55] Replacing MR imaging with CT in PET/MR imaging yields a higher detection of these mucinous liver metastases in patients with colorectal carcinoma[56] (**Fig. 9**).

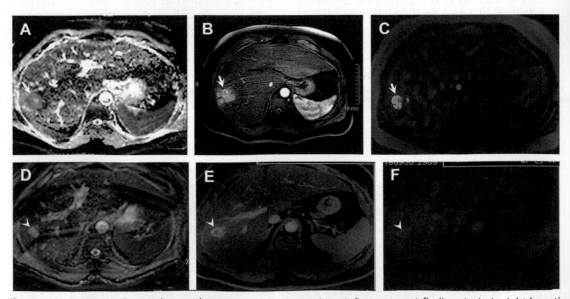

Fig. 6. Liver metastasis from colon carcinoma—response to treatment. Pretreatment findings include right hepatic lobe metastasis (*arrows*) with restricted diffusion as shown by low-signal intensity on ADC map MR image (*A*), enhancement on contrast-enhanced T1-weighted MR image (*B*), and intense FDG uptake on fused hybrid PET/MR image (*C*). Postchemotherapy follow-up findings not only include decrease in size of metastasis (*arrowheads*) but also improvement in diffusion restriction as shown by high signal intensity on ADC map MR image (*D*), minimal enhancement on contrast-enhanced T1-weighted MR image (*E*), and no FDG uptake on fused hybrid PET/MR image (*F*).

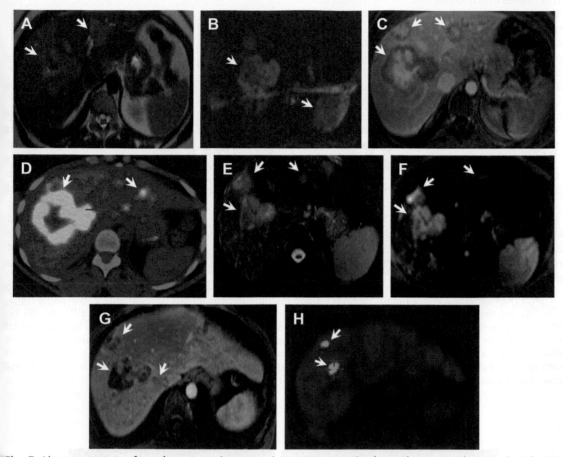

Fig. 7. Liver metastases from breast carcinoma resistant to systemic chemotherapy and treated with 90Y radioembolization. Pretreatment findings include hepatic metastases (*arrows*) in right and left hepatic lobes with hyperintense T2-weighted signal intensity relative to liver (*A*), restricted diffusion (*B*), enhancement on contrast-enhanced T1-weighted image (*C*) on MR imaging, and intense FDG uptake on PET/CT image (*D*). Post-90Y radioembolization findings include decrease in size of lesions (*arrows*) with persistent hyperintense T2-weighted signal intensity (*E*) and restricted diffusion (*F*) secondary to posttreatment edema, inflammation, or fibrosis but with decreased enhancement on contrast-enhanced T1-weighted image (*G*) on MR imaging and improved FDG uptake with residual small foci of FDG uptake seen on fused PET/MR image (*H*), indicating good response to locoregional therapy with persistent residual disease.

Cholangiocarcinoma

Cholangiocarcinoma is a malignancy of the biliary tract that has increased in incidence over time and represents the second most common primary hepatic malignancy.[57] Cholangio-carcinomas are extremely difficult to diagnose and pose a diagnostic and therapeutic challenge owing to different histologic types, growth patterns, and clinical manifestations. Usually, patients present late in the disease course, which in combination with difficulty of diagnosis by routine imaging, results in high mortality.[58–60]

Morphologically, these tumors are categorized into exophytic mass forming, periductal infiltrating, and intraductal polypoid or infiltrating types. The peripheral mass forming cholangio-carcinoma is well identified by both contrast-enhanced CT and MR imaging owing to its characteristic initial peripheral rim enhancement with gradual centripetal enhancement on delayed phase images. It may be associated with peripheral ductal dilation. Periductal infiltrating cholangiocarcinomas and those seen in the setting of primary sclerosing cholangitis without a distinct mass are difficult to detect by contrast-enhanced CT. MR imaging with magnetic resonance cholangiopancreatography (MRCP) and delayed-phase contrast-enhanced MR images have higher sensitivity in depicting these tumors at the site of biliary stricture.[61,62]

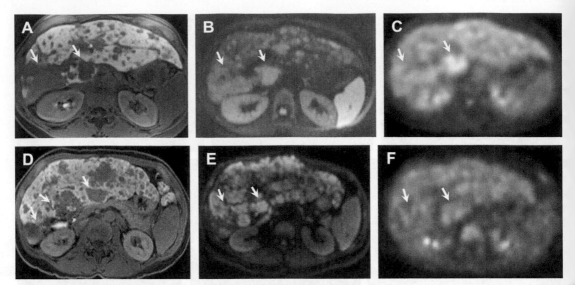

Fig. 8. Post-90Y radioembolization follow-up of diffuse liver metastases from breast carcinoma resistant to systemic chemotherapy. Pretreatment findings include multiple hepatic lesions (*arrows*) with hypointense signal intensity on hepatobiliary phase contrast-enhanced T1-weighted images (*A*) and restricted diffusion (*B*) on MR imaging and variable degrees of FDG uptake on PET images (*C*). Post-90Y treatment findings include interval decrease in size of multiple hepatic lesions (*arrows*) again with hypointense signal intensity on hepatobiliary phase contrast-enhanced T1-weighted image (*D*) and less restricted diffusion (*E*) on MR imaging and decreased FDG uptake of dominant lesions on PET images (*F*). Because of pseudocirrhosis of liver, FDG PET was more useful than MR imaging for assessment of tumor response to treatment.

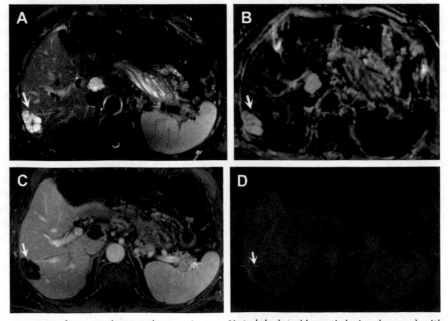

Fig. 9. Liver metastases form mucinous colon carcinoma. Note lobulated hepatic lesion (*arrows*) with central scar, thin septations, and hyperintense signal intensity relative to liver on T2-weighted MR image (*A*), predominantly cystic appearance except for internal septa on ADC map MR image (*B*), and central enhancing scar and thin septations on contrast-enhanced T1-weighted MR image (*C*). Fused PET/MR image (*D*) shows no FDG uptake in lesion (*arrow*). FDG PET provided a false-negative result, but MR imaging findings were useful to differentiate this metastasis from a hepatic cyst.

There is paucity of literature highlighting the role of PET/CT in assessing these tumors, but it has been found that FDG uptake depends on morphologic characteristics and location of the lesions, with peripheral mass-forming lesions showing more avid FDG uptake, which are hence better detected than periductal infiltrating and hilar lesions.[63–65] Low FDG uptake in the periductal infiltrating type is caused by small tumor volume with more fibrous stroma and low cellularity. False-negative results are also seen in predominantly mucinous cholangiocarcinomas, which are usually non-FDG avid.[61,66] FDG PET faces similar challenges to contrast-enhanced MR imaging in differentiating benign from malignant biliary strictures, as increased FDG uptake can also be seen in benign strictures owing to inflammation secondary to stent placement or from primary sclerosing cholangitis.[67,68] Kim and colleagues[59] found FDG PET/CT offers no advantage over contrast-enhanced CT, MR imaging, or MRCP in diagnosing primary biliary tumors but improves detection of regional nodal and distant metastases. The diagnostic accuracies for nodal detection for FDG PET, CT, and MR imaging in this study were 86%, 68%, and 57%, respectively.

Although there is no substantive data on role of FDG PET/MR imaging, our initial experience suggests that PET/MR imaging has an advantage over PET/CT or MR imaging alone in initial detection of primary cholangiocarcinoma, although the true potential of this new modality has yet to be explored. It has a potential role in initial staging, for assessment of treatment response, and also in follow up after treatment, especially in patients with peripheral mass forming cholangiocarcinoma[69,70] (**Fig. 10**).

Gallbladder Cancer

Gallbladder cancer is the fifth most common GI malignancy and the most common malignancy of the biliary tree with nonspecific clinical presentation and aggressive biologic characteristics, contributing to advanced stage and dismal prognosis at the time of initial presentation.[71] Because of the elusive nature of this cancer, only less than 10% are resectable, and nearly 50% have associated lymph nodal metastases.[72]

Advanced gallbladder cancers are relatively easy to detect, but imaging detection at early stages remain elusive, mainly because of considerable overlap between benign entities like chronic cholecystitis and early malignancy, both producing gallbladder wall thickening. In many cases, MR imaging is helpful in making this distinction, with typical imaging features of asymmetric and

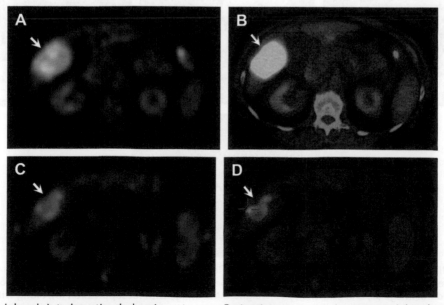

Fig. 10. Peripheral intrahepatic cholangiocarcinoma. Pretreatment study shows a peripheral well-defined segment 6 hepatic mass (*arrow*) with restricted diffusion on DW MR image (*A*) and intense FDG uptake (*arrow*) on corresponding PET/CT image (*B*). Postchemotherapy study shows not only decreased size of lesion (*arrow*) with improved restricted diffusion on DW MR image (*C*) but also decreased FDG uptake in lesion (*arrow*) on fused PET/MR image (*D*) indicating good response to treatment.

irregular mural thickening and marked arterial phase enhancement without washout on venous phase images.[73–75] MR imaging combined with MRCP and contrast-enhanced imaging has been reported to be up to 100% sensitive for detecting bile duct and vascular invasion, although the sensitivity for hepatic invasion and lymph node involvement is only 67% and 56%, respectively.[63,76]

Until now, only a handful of studies assessed the role of FDG PET/CT in gallbladder cancer. Recent studies found that PET/CT has the potential to improve detection of primary and metastatic gallbladder malignancies.[63,77] Oe and colleagues[78]

found that increased FDG uptake can be helpful in distinguishing between benign and malignant gallbladder wall thickening, seen on ultrasonography, CT, or MR imaging (**Fig. 11**). Nishiyama and colleagues[79] reported that delayed time point FDG PET imaging can improve lesion detection by increasing the degree of radiotracer uptake in lesions and improving the target to background contrast. FDG PET is found to be more useful in detection of nodal and extrahepatic metastases and in follow-up evaluation for postsurgical recurrence[80,81] (**Fig. 12**).

However, prospective studies directly comparing role of MR imaging and PET/CT in

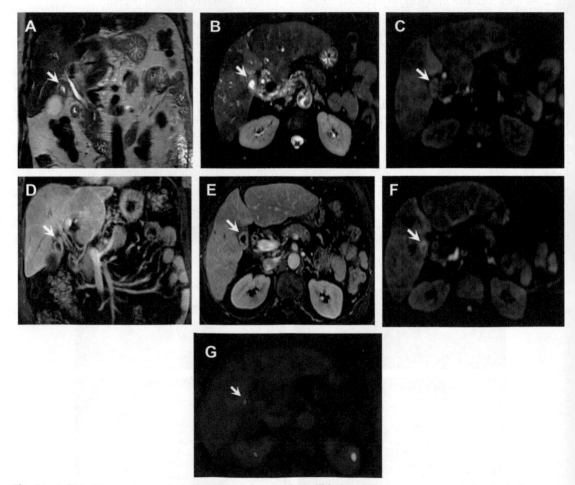

Fig. 11. Gallbladder carcinoma in patient with nonspecific gallbladder distention seen on abdominal ultrasonography. Note focal mural thickening of gallbladder neck (*arrows*) close to cystic duct on coronal heavily T2-weighted MR image (*A*) and axial heavy T2-weighted MR image with fat suppression (*B*), along with enhancement on corresponding coronal (*D*) and axial (*E*) contrast-enhanced T1-weighted MR images. Focal restricted diffusion is also seen in this region (*arrows*) on DW MR images (*C, F*). Fused PET/MR image (*G*) shows focal intense FDG uptake in gallbladder neck (*arrow*). Cholecystectomy found focal adenocarcinoma of gallbladder neck with extension to cystic duct. Hybrid PET/MR imaging was useful to detect gallbladder carcinoma and to plan treatment in this patient who had presented with nonspecific symptoms and ultrasonographic findings (not shown).

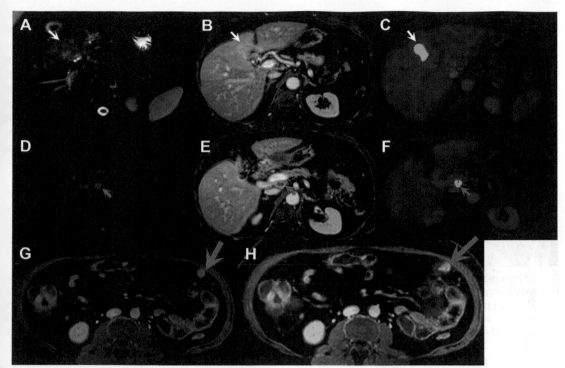

Fig. 12. Gallbladder carcinoma—post-surgical recurrence 1 year after prior cholecystectomy. Note ill-defined mass (*arrows*) in segment 4B of liver with hyperintense signal intensity on T2-weighted MR image (*A*), enhancement on contrast-enhanced T1-weighted MR image (*B*), and intense FDG uptake on fused PET/MR image (*C*). Axial DWI (*D*) and contrast-enhanced (*E*) MR images show an enlarged portacaval lymph node (*yellow arrows*) with intense FDG uptake on fused PET/MR image (*F*) owing to nodal metastatic disease. Axial contrast-enhanced T1-weighted MR image (*G*) and corresponding fused PET/MR image (*H*) show an FDG-avid peritoneal implant (*large arrows*). Hybrid PET/MR imaging was useful in this patient to detect not only local recurrence in the liver but also to identify extrahepatic nodal and peritoneal metastases.

gallbladder malignancies have not been performed. The role of PET/MR imaging in initial staging of gallbladder carcinoma has yet to be established. Better tissue characterization and delineation of biliary anatomy with MR imaging and FDG PET evaluation of the whole body suggests PET/MR imaging may be better than PET/CT for TNM staging of gallbladder cancer and may have a positive impact on therapy selection.

Pancreatic Carcinoma

Contrast-enhanced CT is the initial imaging method for evaluation of patients suspected to have pancreatic cancer. Both contrast-enhanced CT and MR imaging have similar accuracy in the detection of pancreatic carcinoma and assessment of local extension and resectability.[82,83] However, contrast-enhanced CT has limited sensitivity in detection of hepatic and peritoneal metastases.[84] Contrast-enhanced

MR imaging is used as an alternative imaging method when equivocal findings are detected on contrast-enhanced CT. This finding occurs often when no discrete pancreatic mass is identified on CT or when characterization of indeterminate liver lesions is required to exclude metastases.[85] The value of FDG PET in initial diagnosis of pancreatic carcinoma is not defined. This finding is caused by to the high sensitivity and accuracy of CT and MR imaging in pancreatic carcinoma detection and T staging. Both CT and MR imaging have relatively low sensitivity in detection of nodal and distant metastases. FDG PET/CT has low sensitivity of 30% to 49% in the detection of nodal metastases but has a higher sensitivity of up to 88% and an accuracy of 94% in the detection of distant metastases[83] (**Fig. 13**).

Most of the available PET/MR imaging literature regarding pancreatic disease is based on retrospective fusion of PET and MR imaging

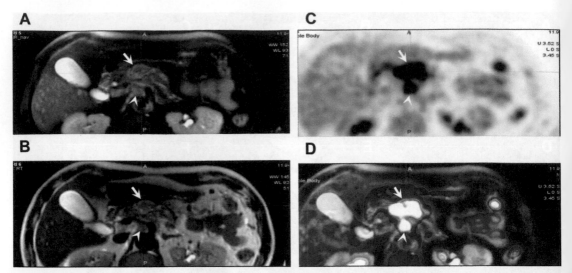

Fig. 13. Pancreatic carcinoma—staging. Note pancreatic head mass (*arrows*) and enlarged preaortic retroperitoneal lymph node (*arrowheads*) on T2-weighted MR images with (*A*) and without (*B*) fat suppression as well as avid FDG uptake in pancreatic mass (*arrows*) and preaortic retroperitoneal lymph node (*arrowheads*) on PET image (*C*) and fused PET/MR image (*D*). The good soft tissue contrast resolution of MR imaging was helpful to separate the primary pancreatic mass from an adjacent lymph node for proper staging and treatment planning.

data. Tatsumi and colleagues[86] assessed the feasibility of retrospective PET and MR imaging fusion and found an advantage of combining PET images with noncontrast T1-weighted MR images over PET/CT in the characterization of pancreatic tumors. Nagamachi and colleagues[87] found significantly improved accuracy in differentiating pancreatic cancer from benign lesions using retrospectively fused PET and T2-weighted MR images compared with PET/CT (96.6% vs 86.6%, respectively). Additionally, T2-weighted images provide much better demonstration of the internal architecture of pancreatic cystic lesions, helping to differentiate benign cysts from malignant cystic neoplasms. Retrospective fusion has an unavoidable limitation of misregistration of the data owing to the temporal differences in data acquisition.

PET/MR imaging has a selective role in the initial imaging of those patients with suspected carcinoma with a pancreatic duct stricture in which no distinct mass is visualized on contrast-enhanced CT. Combination of MR imaging with MRCP and FDG PET has ability to identify small mass lesions at the stricture site and to direct endoscopic ultrasound-guided biopsy. The combination of MR imaging with DWI and FDG PET has an advantage over both contrast-enhanced CT and PET/CT in the detection of early hepatic metastases and to

avoid unnecessary surgery. Both CT and FDG PET have low sensitivity and accuracy for detection of peritoneal implants, another major factor affecting surgical resectability. MR imaging with DWI as part of PET/MR imaging has better sensitivity in detection of peritoneal implants.[88,89] Detection of tumor recurrence after surgery is challenging with CT owing to altered anatomy and high false-negative and false-positive rates. Several studies found FDG PET to have higher accuracy in the detection of local recurrence of pancreatic carcinoma.[90,91] Better anatomic delineation of the surgical bed by MR imaging and metabolic information from FDG activity via PET/MR imaging are promising for optimized detection of local tumor recurrence (**Fig. 14**).

The approach to diagnosis of gastroenteropancreatic neuroendocrine tumors has significantly changed with the introduction of new radiotracers labeled with 68Ga.[92,93] Several PET/CT studies found higher accuracy and better lesion detection with 68Ga-labeled radiotracers. A recent simultaneous PET/MR imaging pilot study by Beiderwellen and colleagues[94] in patients with gastroenteropancreatic neuroendocrine tumors using 68Ga-DOTA-D-Phe1-Tyr3-octreotide (68Ga-DOTATOC) found advantages in characterization of abdominal lesions using PET/MR imaging when compared with 68Ga-DOTATOC PET/CT.

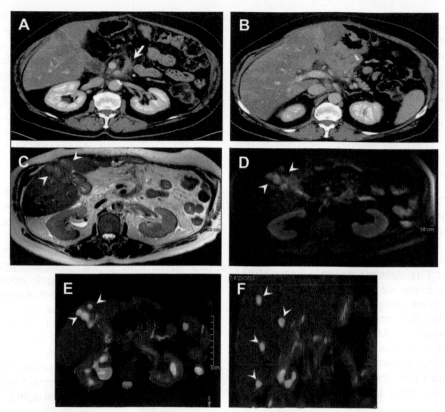

Fig. 14. Pancreatic carcinoma follow-up evaluation after Whipple procedure for increasing serum CA-19-9 levels and suspicious local recurrence on contrast-enhanced CT. Axial contrast-enhanced CT images (*A, B*) show nonspecific soft tissue haziness in surgical bed near superior mesenteric vessels (*arrow*). Follow-up assessment shows no mass in the surgical bed on T2-weighted (*C*) and axial DWI (*D*) MR images but shows multiple hepatic lesions (*arrowheads*) with high T2-weighted signal intensity and restricted diffusion. Intense FDG uptake is also present in the hepatic lesions (*arrowheads*) on fused PET/MR images (*E, F*). These findings are in keeping with metastases. The better soft tissue contrast of MR imaging was helpful to evaluate the surgical bed, whereas combined PET/MR imaging was able to detect liver metastases missed on CT, which accounted for the increase in serum CA-19-9 levels.

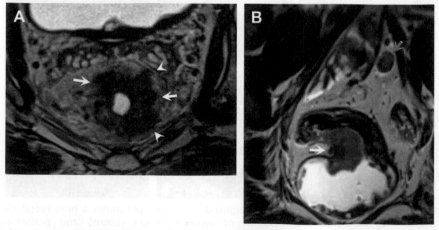

Fig. 15. Rectal carcinoma—staging. High-resolution T2-weighted MR images in axial (*A*) and coronal (*B*) planes show a rectal mass with transmural invasion into perirectal fat (*arrows*) with good delineation of tumor extension to the mesorectal fascia (*arrowheads*), along with an enlarged superior rectal lymph node (*yellow arrow*) with heterogeneous signal intensity. High-resolution T2-weighted MR images are an essential component of PET/MR imaging in T staging of rectal carcinoma, which is advantageous compared with the low soft tissue contrast resolution of CT in PET/CT.

Colorectal Cancer

CT of the chest, abdomen, and pelvis is recommended for the initial preoperative assessment of patients with colorectal carcinoma. MR imaging is an accepted modality for staging of rectal cancer, allowing an accurate identification of transmural invasion of the mesorectal fat and mesorectal fascia involvement by tumor (**Fig. 15**).[95,96] CT significantly lacks soft tissue contrast resolution so that its utility in T staging of rectal cancer is limited. Because of the higher sensitivity and specificity compared with CT, FDG PET/CT is recommended for use in the metastatic workup for colorectal cancer and has been found to improve lesion localization and diagnostic confidence compared with FDG PET imaging alone.[97,98] In treatment monitoring and follow-up, CT is valuable because of its ability to delineate tumor size and visceral involvement and has been adopted to measure tumor response by Response Evaluation Criteria in Solid Tumors.[99,100] MR imaging has proven to be valuable to assess local therapy response[101] and to restage colorectal cancer.[102] FDG PET seems to be better than CT and MR imaging in predicting response to preoperative therapy of locally advanced rectal cancer.[103] In a study comparing FDG PET/CT with whole-body MR imaging at 1.5 T and 3 T in patients with recurrent colorectal cancer, PET/CT was found to be more accurate than MR imaging in lymph node metastases (sensitivity, 93% vs 63%, respectively). Both modalities had similar sensitivity for the detection of organ metastases (sensitivity, 78% for PET and 80% for MR imaging).[104] The overall diagnostic accuracy was 91% for PET/CT (sensitivity, 86%; specificity, 96%) and 83% for MR imaging (sensitivity, 72%; specificity, 93%).[104] Nonetheless, FDG PET/CT had limited accuracy in the detection of small liver lesions, which were better depicted with MR imaging.[105]

Considering the aforementioned complementary advantages of PET and MR imaging, the use of a hybrid PET/MR imaging could serve as a one-stop imaging approach that potentially improves diagnostic confidence and accuracy in colorectal cancer (**Fig. 16**). In colon carcinoma, replacement of CT with MR imaging in hybrid FDG PET imaging has the advantage of characterization of liver lesions and detection of small metastases, which has an impact on treatment planning. Use of liver-specific contrast-

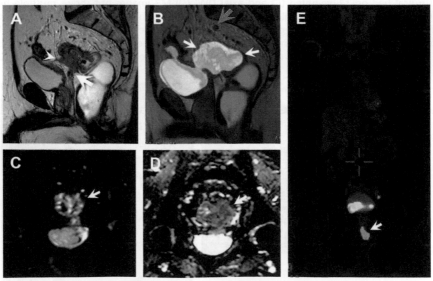

Fig. 16. Rectal carcinoma—staging. Sagittal T2-weighted MR image (A) shows a high rectal circumferential mass with transmural extension and invasion of seminal vesicle (*arrow*) and peritoneal reflection (*arrowhead*). Axial DWI (C) and ADC map (D) MR images show restricted diffusion of rectal mass. Fused hybrid PET/MR imaging sagittal image (B) shows intense FDG uptake of rectal mass (*arrows*) with no uptake in a superior rectal lymph node (*yellow arrow*). Whole-body fused coronal PET/MR image (E) shows FDG-avid rectal mass (*arrow*) and no evidence of distant metastases. Hybrid PET/MR imaging has a potential use as a 1-stop single imaging technique for staging of locally advanced rectal carcinoma and for treatment planning.

enhanced MR imaging has improved detection of small hepatic metastases. In rectal carcinoma, PET/MR imaging has the advantage of high-resolution MR imaging in determining the T stage of rectal cancer.[95,96] Neither PET scanning at PET/MR imaging nor PET/CT scanning provides additional relevant information to T staging besides MR imaging. PET/MR imaging is expected to be more accurate than PET/CT in N and M staging as well considering the high soft tissue

contrast provided by MR imaging compared with CT,[102] but future research is warranted in this regard. Initial experience from a pilot study shows high accuracy of the combined PET/MR imaging in T staging of colorectal carcinoma compared with PET/CT with at least comparable accuracy in N and M staging.[106] MR imaging with DWI is of added value in predicting the response of rectal carcinoma to neoadjuvant treatment and in identifying the degree of tumor

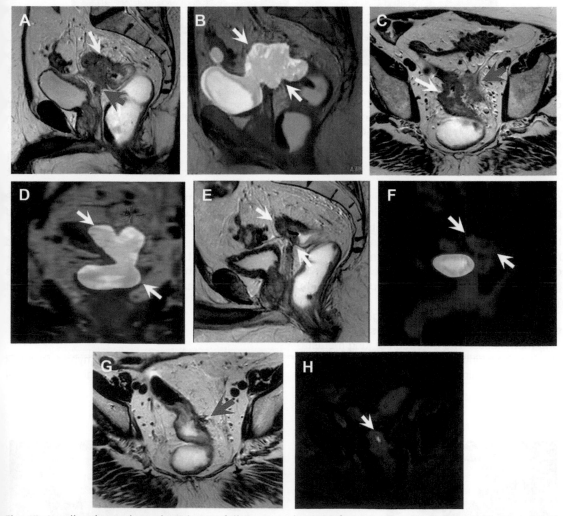

Fig. 17. Locally advanced rectal carcinoma follow-up evaluation after neoadjuvant chemoradiation treatment. Pretreatment hybrid PET/MR images of same patient as in **Fig. 16** again show high rectal circumferential mass (*arrows*) with transmural invasion (*yellow arrow*) on sagittal (*A*) and axial (*C*) T2-weighted MR images and intense FDG uptake on fused sagittal (*B*) and coronal PET/MR (*D*) images. Posttreatment hybrid PET/MR images show not only significant decrease in tumor size (*arrows*) including extramural extension (*yellow arrow*) on T2-weighted MR images (*E, G*) but also marked decrease in FDG uptake on fused PET/MR images (*F, H*) indicating near complete response. Hybrid PET/MR imaging with combined anatomic (T2-weighted MR imaging), functional (DWI), and metabolic (FDG PET) information is useful to assess treatment response of rectal carcinoma after neoadjuvant chemoradiation treatment.

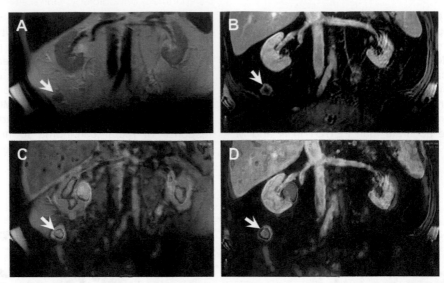

Fig. 18. Follow-up evaluation of resected sigmoid colon carcinoma for increasing serum carcinoembryonic anti-gen levels. Hybrid PET/MR images show peritoneal nodule (*arrows*) on coronal T2-weighted (*A*) and coronal contrast-enhanced T1-weighted (*B*) MR images, along with intense FDG uptake on corresponding coronal fused PET/MR images (*C, D*). No other metastases were seen on whole-body PET/MR images. PET/MR imaging can be an alternative to PET/CT in selected patients for surveillance of treated colon carcinoma with increasing serum car-cinoembryonic antigen levels.

response after treatment.[107–109] FDG PET provides additional metabolic information in addition to morphologic and functional informa-tion from MR imaging to assess treatment response after neoadjuvant treatment of rectal carcinoma and to detect and localize postsur-gical recurrence of colorectal carcinoma (**Figs. 17** and **18**).[103]

Both FDG PET and MR imaging have low sensitivity in the detection of less than 1 cm lung metastases. The detection of lung metasta-ses can be significantly improved by adding a diagnostic 3-dimensional contrast-enhanced

T1-weighted imaging sequence to the PET/MR imaging protocol. Because the detection rate of small lung metastases is still inferior to PET/CT and diagnostic CT of the chest, an unenhanced CT of the chest may be considered after a nega-tive PET/MR imaging for lung metastases if it is going to change the patient management (**Fig. 19**).[110,111]

SUMMARY

The initial clinical experience of hybrid PET/MR imaging is promising in oncologic diseases of

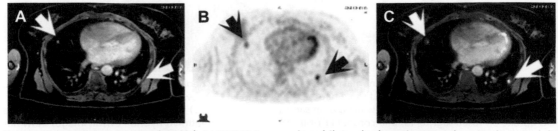

Fig. 19. Colon carcinoma—staging. Hybrid PET/MR images show bilateral subcentimeter-enhancing lung nodules (*arrows*) on axial T1-weighted MR image (*A*) with FDG uptake on PET image (*B*) and fused PET/MR image (*C*). PET/MR imaging is limited for detection of subcentimeter lung metastases owing to low sensitivity of both MR imaging and FDG PET compared with CT. However, contrast-enhanced T1-weighted MR imaging is useful for detection of lung metastases.

the GI tract. PET/CT is a well-established hybrid PET imaging technique for staging and follow-up of patients with GI tract malignancies, especially for colorectal carcinoma. PET/MR imaging is not going to replace PET/CT, but it is found to be useful wherever the high soft tissue contrast resolution of MR imaging has an advantage over CT such as in rectal carcinoma and for the characterization of liver lesions. Functional MR imaging techniques such as DWI add to the metabolic information from FDG PET in more accurate assessment of tumor response and local recurrence after treatment of colorectal carcinoma. The role of PET/MR imaging in detection and follow-up of HCC is limited with FDG, and the advent of new radiotracers may improve its utility. Approval of 68Ga-DOTATOC for clinical use will also further increase the role of PET/MR imaging in staging and follow-up of neuroendocrine tumors. Based on the current preliminary data, PET/MR imaging with FDG has clinical utility in selected patients with GI tract malignancy for initial staging and for follow-up evaluation after systemic and locoregional treatment.

REFERENCES

1. Antoch G, Bockisch A. Combined PET/MRI: a new dimension in whole-body oncology imaging? Eur J Nucl Med Mol Imaging 2009;36(Suppl 1):S113–20.
2. Balyasnikova S, Löfgren J, de Nijs R, et al. PET/MR in oncology: an introduction with focus on MR and future perspectives for hybrid imaging. Am J Nucl Med Mol Imaging 2012;2:458–74.
3. Zaidi H, Montandon ML, Alavi A. The clinical role of fusion imaging using PET, CT, and MR imaging. Magn Reson Imaging Clin N Am 2010;18:133–49.
4. Schöder H, Larson SM, Yeung HWD. PET/CT in oncology: integration into clinical management of lymphoma, melanoma, and gastrointestinal malignancies. J Nucl Med 2004;45(Suppl 1):72S–81S.
5. von Schulthess GK, Steinert HC, Hany TF. Integrated PET/CT: current applications and future directions. Radiology 2006;238:405–22.
6. Drzezga A, Souvatzoglou M, Eiber M, et al. First Clinical experience with integrated whole-body PET/MR: comparison to PET/CT in patients with oncologic diagnoses. J Nucl Med 2012;53:845–55.
7. Catalano OA, Rosen BR, Sahani DV, et al. Clinical impact of PET/MR imaging in patients with cancer undergoing same-day PET/CT: initial experience in 134 patients–a hypothesis-generating exploratory study. Radiology 2013;269:857–69.
8. Czernin J, Ta L, Herrmann K. Does PET/MR imaging improve cancer assessments? literature evidence from more than 900 patients. J Nucl Med 2014;55(Suppl 2):59S–62S.
9. Delso G, Ziegler S. PET/MRI system design. Eur J Nucl Med Mol Imaging 2009;36(suppl 1):S86–92.
10. Herzog H, Van Den Hoff J. Combined PET/MR systems: an overview and comparison of currently available options. Q J Nucl Med Mol Imaging 2012;56:247–67.
11. Torigian DA, Zaidi H, Kwee TC, et al. PET/MR imaging: technical aspects and potential clinical applications. Radiology 2013;267:26–44.
12. Vaska P, Cao T. The state of instrumentation for combined positron emission tomography and magnetic resonance imaging. Semin Nucl Med 2013;43:11–8.
13. Lecomte R, Cadorette J, Rodrigue S, et al. Initial results from the sherbrooke avalanche photodiode positron tomograph. IEEE Trans Nucl Sci 1996;43:1952–7.
14. Yoon HS, Ko GB, Kwon S, et al. Initial results of simultaneous PET/MRI experiments with an MRI-compatible siliconphotomultiplier PET scanner. J Nucl Med 2012;53:608–14.
15. Yankeelov TE, Peterson TE, Abramson RG, et al. Simultaneous PET-MRI in oncology: a solution looking for a problem? Magn Reson Imaging 2012;30:1342–56.
16. Yoo HJ, Lee JS, Lee JM. Integrated whole body MR/PET: where are we? Korean J Radiol 2015;16(1):32–49.
17. Werner M, Schmidt H, Schwenzer N. MR/PET: a new challenge in hybrid imaging. Am J Roentgenol 2012;199:272.
18. Bagade S, Fowler KJ, Schwarz JK, et al. PET/MRI evaluation of gynecologic malignancies and prostate cancer. Semin Nucl Med 2015 Jul;45(4):293–303.
19. Gu J, Chan T, Zhang J, et al. Whole-body diffusion-weighted imaging: the added value to whole-body MRI at initial diagnosis of lymphoma. AJR Am J Roentgenol 2011;197(3):W384–91.
20. Abdulqadhr G, Molin D, Aström G, et al. Whole-body diffusion-weighted imaging compared with FDG-PET/CT in staging of lymphoma patients. Acta Radiol 2011;52:173–80.
21. Siegel MJ, Acharyya S, Hoffer FA, et al. Whole-Body MR imaging for staging of malignant tumors in pediatric patients: results of the American College of Radiology Imaging Network 6660 Trial. Radiology 2013;266(2):599–609.
22. Partovi S, Kohan A, Rubbert C, et al. Clinical oncologic applications of PET/MRI: a new horizon. Am J Nucl Med Mol Imaging 2014;4(2):202–12.
23. Fraum TJ, Fowler KJ, McConathy J, et al. PET/MRI for the body imager: abdominal and pelvic oncologic applications. Abdom Imaging 2015;40(6):1387–404.

24. Sugita R, Ito K, Fujita N, et al. Diffusion-weighted MRI in abdominal oncology: clinical applications. World J Gastroenterol 2010;16(7):832–6.

25. Vandecaveye V, De Keyzer F, Vander Poorten V, et al. Head and neck squamous cell carcinoma: value of diffusion-weighted MR imaging for nodal staging. Radiology 2009;251:134–46.

26. Fujii S, Matsusue E, Kanasaki Y, et al. Detection of peritoneal dissemination in gynecological malignancy: evaluation by diffusion-weighted MR imaging. Eur Radiol 2008;18(1):18–23.

27. Waghray A, Murali AR, Menon KN. Hepatocellular carcinoma: from diagnosis to treatment. World J Hepatol 2015;7(8):1020–9.

28. Schima W, Hammerstingl R, Catalano C, et al. Quadruple-phase MDCT of the liver in patients with suspected hepatocellular carcinoma: effect of contrast material flow rate. AJR Am J Roentgenol 2006;186(6):1571–9.

29. Kim SK, Lim JH, Lee WJ, et al. Detection of hepatocellular carcinoma: comparison of dynamic three-phase computed tomography images and four-phase computed tomography images using multidetector row helical computed tomography. J Comput Assist Tomogr 2002;26(5):691–8.

30. Piana G, Trinquart L, Meskine N, et al. New MR imaging criteria with a diffusion-weighted sequence for the diagnosis of hepatocellular carcinoma in chronic liver diseases. J Hepatol 2011; 55(1):126–32.

31. Yu JS, Chung JJ, Kim JH, et al. Detection of small intrahepatic metastases of hepatocellular carcinomas using diffusion-weighted imaging: comparison with conventional dynamic MRI. Magn Reson Imaging 2011;29:985–92.

32. Di Martino M, Marin D, Guerrisi A, et al. Intraindividual comparison of gadoxetate disodium-enhanced MR imaging and 64-section multidetector CT in the detection of hepatocellular carcinoma in patients with cirrhosis. Radiology 2010;256:806–16.

33. Park G, Kim YK, Kim CS, et al. Diagnostic efficacy of gadoxetic acid-enhanced MRI in the detection of hepatocellular carcinomas: comparison with gadopentetate dimeglumine. Br J Radiol 2010;83: 1010–6.

34. Holalkere NS, Sahani DV, Blake MA, et al. Characterization of small liver lesions: added value of MR after MDCT. J Comput Assist Tomogr 2006; 30:591–6.

35. Wudel LJ Jr, Delbeke D, Morris D, et al. The role of [18F]fluorodeoxyglucose positron emission tomography imaging in the evaluation of hepatocellular carcinoma. Am Surg 2003;69(2):117–24 [discussion: 124–6].

36. Wolfort RM, Papillion PW, Turnage RH, et al. Role of FDG-PET in the evaluation and staging of hepatocellular carcinoma with comparison of tumor size, AFP level, and histologic grade. Int Surg 2010; 95(1):67–75.

37. Park JW, Kim JH, Kim SK, et al. A prospective evaluation of 18F-FDG and 11C-acetate PET/CT for detection of primary and metastatic hepatocellular carcinoma. J Nucl Med 2008;49: 1912–21.

38. Talbot JN, Fartoux L, Balogova S, et al. Detection of hepatocellular carcinoma with PET/CT: a prospective comparison of 18F- fluorocholine and18F-FDG in patients with cirrhosis or chronic liver disease. J Nucl Med 2010;51:1699–706.

39. Song MJ, Bae SH, Lee SW, et al. 18F-fluorodeoxyglucose PET/CT predicts tumour progression after transarterial chemoembolization in hepatocellular carcinoma. Eur J Nucl Med Mol Imaging 2013; 40(6):865–73.

40. Huang WY, Kao CH, Huang WS, et al. 18F-FDG PET and combined 18F-FDG-contrast CT parameters as predictors of tumor control for hepatocellular carcinoma after stereotactic ablative radiotherapy. J Nucl Med 2013;54(10):1710–6.

41. Sugiyama M, Sakahara H, Torizuka T, et al. 18F-FDG PET in the detection of extrahepatic metastases from hepatocellular carcinoma. J Gastroenterol 2004;39(10):961–8.

42. Yoon KT, Kim JK, Kim do Y, et al. Role of 18F-fluorodeoxyglucose positron emission tomography in detecting extrahepatic metastasis in pretreatment staging of hepatocellular carcinoma. Oncology 2007;72(Suppl 1):104–10.

43. Beiderwellen K, Geraldo L, Ruhlmann V, et al. Accuracy of [18F]FDG PET/MRI for the detection of liver metastases. PLoS One 2015;10(9): e0137285.

44. Seo HJ, Kim MJ, Lee JD, et al. Gadoxetate disodium-enhanced magnetic resonance imaging versus contrast-enhanced 18F-fluorodeoxyglucose positron emission tomography/computed tomography for the detection of colorectal liver metastases. Invest Radiol 2011;46(9):548–55.

45. Donati OF, Hany TF, Reiner CS, et al. Value of retrospective fusion of PET and MR images in detection of hepatic metastases: comparison with 18F-FDG PET/CT and Gd-EOB-DTPA-enhanced MRI. J Nucl Med 2010;51(5):692–9.

46. Kwee TC, Takahara T, Ochiai R, et al. Diffusion-weighted whole-body imaging with background body signal suppression (DWIBS): features and potential applications in oncology. Eur Radiol 2008;18:1937–52.

47. Klerkx WM, Geldof AA, Heintz AP, et al. Longitudinal 3.0T MRI analysis of changes in lymph node volume and apparent diffusion coefficient in an experimental animal model of metastatic and hyperplastic lymph nodes. J Magn Reson Imaging 2011;33:1151–9.

48. Lee JW, Paeng JC, Kang KW, et al. Prediction of tumor recurrence by 18F-FDG PET in liver transplantation for hepatocellular carcinoma. J Nucl Med 2009;50(5):682–7.

49. Sheth KR, Clary BM. Management of hepatic metastases from colorectal cancer. Clin Colon Rectal Surg 2005;18(3):215–23.

50. Kelly H, Goldberg RM. Systemic therapy for metastatic colorectal cancer: current options, current evidence. J Clin Oncol 2005;23(20):4553–60.

51. Mainenti PP, Mancini M, Mainolfi C, et al. Detection of colo-rectal liver metastases: prospective comparison of contrast enhanced US, multidetector CT, PET/CT, and 1.5 Tesla MR with extracellular and reticulo-endothelial cell specific contrast agents. Abdom Imaging 2010;35(5):511–21.

52. Yong TW, Yuan ZZ, Jun Z, et al. Sensitivity of PET/MR images in liver metastases from colorectal carcinoma. Hell J Nucl Med 2011;14(3):264–8.

53. Reiner CS, Stolzmann P, Husmann L, et al. Protocol requirements and diagnostic value of PET/MR imaging for liver metastasis detection. Eur J Nucl Med Mol Imaging 2014;41(4):649–58.

54. Berger KL, Nicholson SA, Dehdashti F, et al. FDG PET evaluation of mucinous neoplasms: correlation of FDG uptake with histopathologic features. AJR Am J Roentgenol 2000;174(4):1005–8.

55. Whiteford MH, Whiteford HM, Yee LF, et al. Usefulness of FDG-PET scan in the assessment of suspected metastatic or recurrent adenocarcinoma of the colon and rectum. Dis Colon Rectum 2000; 43(6):759–67.

56. Lee DH, Lee JM, Hur BY, et al. Colorectal cancer liver metastases: diagnostic performance and prognostic value of PET/MR Imaging. Radiology 2016;19:151975.

57. Cai Y, Cheng N, Ye H, et al. The current management of cholangiocarcinoma: a comparison of current guidelines. Biosci Trends 2016;10:92–102.

58. Ishak KG, Anthony PP, Sobin LH. Histological typing of tumours of the liver: WHO international histological classification of tumours. Berlin: Springer-Verlag; 1994.

59. Kim JY, Kim MH, Lee TY, et al. Clinical role of 18F-FDG PET-CT in suspected and potentially operable cholangiocarcinoma: a prospective study compared with conventional imaging. Am J Gastroenterol 2008;103(5):1145–51.

60. Singh P, Patel T. Advances in the diagnosis, evaluation and management of cholangiocarcinoma. Curr Opin Gastroenterol 2006;22(3):294–9.

61. Sainani NI, Catalano OA, Holalkere NS, et al. Cholangiocarcinoma: current and novel imaging techniques. Radiographics 2008;28(5):1263–87.

62. Mansfield JC, Griffin SM, Wadehra V, et al. A prospective evaluation of cytology from biliary strictures. Gut 1997;40:671–7.

63. Sacks A, Peller PJ, Surasi DS, et al. Value of PET/CT in the management of primary hepatobiliary tumors, part 2. AJR Am J Roentgenol 2011;197(2): W260–5.

64. Anderson CD, Rice MH, Pinson CW, et al. Fluorodeoxyglucose PET imaging in the evaluation of gallbladder carcinoma and cholangiocarcinoma. J Gastrointest Surg 2004;8:90–7.

65. Nakeeb A, Pitt HA, Sohn TA, et al. Cholangiocarcinoma: a spectrum of intrahepatic, perihilar, and distal tumors. Ann Surg 1996;224:463–73 [discussion: 473–5].

66. Fritscher-Ravens A, Bohuslavizki KH, Broering DC, et al. FDG PET in the diagnosis of hilar cholangiocarcinoma. Nucl Med Commun 2001;22:1277–85.

67. Alkhawaldeh K, Faltten S, Biersack HJ, et al. The value of F-18 FDG PET in patients with primary sclerosing cholangitis and cholangiocarcinoma using visual and semiquantitative analysis. Clin Nucl Med 2011;36(10):879–83.

68. Wakabayashi H, Akamoto S, Yachida S, et al. Significance of fluorodeoxyglucose PET imaging in the diagnosis of malignancies in patients with biliary stricture. Eur J Surg Oncol 2005;31(10): 1175–9.

69. Kim YJ, Yun M, Lee WJ, et al. Usefulness of 18F-FDG PET in intrahepatic cholangiocarcinoma. Eur J Nucl Med Mol Imaging 2003;30(11):1467–72.

70. Jadvar H, Henderson RW, Conti PS. [F-18]fluorodeoxyglucose positron emission tomography and positron emission tomography: computed tomography in recurrent and metastatic cholangiocarcinoma. J Comput Assist Tomogr 2007; 31(2):223–8.

71. Reid KM, Ramos-De la Medina A, Donohue JH. Diagnosis and surgical management of gallbladder cancer: a review. J Gastrointest Surg 2007;11:671–81.

72. Rakić M, Patrlj L, Kopljar M, et al. Gallbladder cancer. Hepatobiliary Surg Nutr 2014;3(5):221–6.

73. Furlan A, Ferris JV, Hosseinzadeh K, et al. Gallbladder carcinoma update: multimodality imaging evaluation, staging, and treatment options. AJR Am J Roentgenol 2008 Nov;191(5):1440–7.

74. Yun EJ, Cho SG, Park S, et al. Gallbladder cancer and chronic cholecystitis: differentiation with two 7phase spiral CT. Abdom Imaging 2004;29:102–8.

75. Yoshimitsu K, Honda H, Kaneko K, et al. Dynamic MRI of the gallbladder lesions: differentiation of benign from malignant. J Magn Reson Imaging 1997;7:696–701.

76. Kim JH, Kim TK, Kim BS, et al. Preoperative evaluation of gallbladder carcinoma: efficacy of combined use of MR imaging, MR cholangiography, and contrast-enhanced dual-phase three-dimensional MR angiography. J Magn Reson Imaging 2002;16:676–84.

77. Ramos-Font C, Gómez Río M, Rodríguez-Fernández A, et al. Positron tomography with 18F-fluorodeoxyglucose in the preoperative evaluation of gall bladder lesions suspicious of malignancy. Diagnostic utility and clinical impact. Rev Esp Med Nucl 2011;30(5):267–75 [in Spanish].

78. Oe A, Kawabe J, Torii K, et al. Distinguishing benign from malignant gallbladder wall thickening using FDG-PET. Ann Nucl Med 2006;20:699–703.

79. Nishiyama Y, Yamamoto Y, Fukunaga K, et al. Dual-time-point 18F-FDG PET for the evaluation of gallbladder carcinoma. J Nucl Med 2006;47:633–8.

80. Lee SW, Kim HJ, Park JH, et al. Clinical usefulness of 18F-FDG PET-CT for patients with gallbladder cancer and cholangiocarcinoma. J Gastroenterol 2010;45(5):560–6.

81. Petrowsky H, Wildbrett P, Husarik DB, et al. Impact of integrated positron emission tomography and computed tomography on staging and management of gallbladder cancer and cholangiocarcinoma. J Hepatol 2006;45(1):43–50.

82. Shrikhande SV, Barreto SG, Goel M, et al. Multimodality imaging of pancreatic ductal adenocarcinoma: a review of the literature. HPB (Oxford) 2012;14(10):658–68.

83. Kauhanen SP, Komar G, Seppänen MP, et al. A prospective diagnostic accuracy study of 18F-fluorodeoxyglucose positron emission tomography/computed tomography, multidetector row computed tomography, and magnetic resonance imaging in primary diagnosis and staging of pancreatic cancer. Ann Surg 2009;250(6):957–63.

84. Wong JC, Lu DS. Staging of pancreatic adenocarcinoma by imaging studies. Clin Gastroenterol Hepatol 2008;6(12):1301–8.

85. Lee ES, Lee JM. Imaging diagnosis of pancreatic cancer: a state-of-the-art review. World J Gastroenterol 2014;20(24):7864–77.

86. Tatsumi M, Isohashi K, Onishi H, et al. 18F-FDG PET/MRI fusion in characterizing pancreatic tumors: comparison to PET/CT. Int J Clin Oncol 2011;16(4):408–15.

87. Nagamachi S, Nishii R, Wakamatsu H, et al. The usefulness of (18)F-FDG PET/MRI fusion image in diagnosing pancreatic tumor: comparison with (18)F-FDG PET/CT. Ann Nucl Med 2013;27(6):554–63.

88. Satoh Y, Ichikawa T, Motosugi U, et al. Diagnosis of peritoneal dissemination: comparison of 18F-FDG PET/CT, diffusion-weighted MRI, and contrast-enhanced MDCT. AJR Am J Roentgenol 2011;196(2):447–53.

89. Soussan M, Des Guetz G, Barrau V, et al. Comparison of FDG-PET/CT and MR with diffusion-weighted imaging for assessing peritoneal carcinomatosis from gastrointestinal malignancy. Eur Radiol 2012;22(7):1479–87.

90. Asagi A, Ohta K, Nasu J, et al. Utility of contrast enhanced FDG-PET/CT in the clinical management of pancreatic cancer: impact on diagnosis, staging, evaluation of treatment response, and detection of recurrence. Pancreas 2013; 42(1):11–9.

91. Hamidian Jahromi A, Sangster G, Zibari G, et al. Accuracy of multi-detector computed tomography, fluorodeoxyglucose positron emission tomography-CT and CA 19-9 levels in detecting recurrent pancreatic adenocarcinoma. JOP 2013;14(4):466–8.

92. Frilling A, Sotiropoulos GC, Radtke A, et al. The impact of 68Ga-DOTATOC positron emission tomography/computed tomography on the multimodal management of patients with neuroendocrine tumors. Ann Surg 2010 Nov;252(5):850–6.

93. Ambrosini V, Campana D, Nanni C, et al. Is ^{68}Ga-DOTA-NOC PET/CT indicated in patients with clinical, biochemical or radiological suspicion of neuroendocrine tumour? Eur J Nucl Med Mol Imaging 2012;39(8):1278–83.

94. Beiderwellen KJ, Poeppel TD, Hartung-Knemeyer V, et al. Simultaneous 68Ga-DOTATOC PET/MRI in patients with gastroenteropancreatic neuroendocrine tumors: initial results. Invest Radiol 2013;48(5):273–9.

95. O'Neill BD, Brown G, Heald RJ, et al. Non-operative treatment after neoadjuvant chemoradiotherapy for rectal cancer. Lancet Oncol 2007;8(7):625–33.

96. Dewhurst CE, Mortele KJ. Magnetic resonance imaging of rectal cancer. Radiol Clin North Am 2013;51(1):121–31.

97. Huebner RH, Park KC, Shepherd JE, et al. A meta-analysis of the literature for whole-body FDG PET detection of recurrent colorectal cancer. J Nucl Med 2000;41(7):1177–89.

98. Cohade C, Osman M, Leal J, et al. Direct comparison of (18)F-FDG PET and PET/CT in patients with colorectal carcinoma. J Nucl Med 2003;44(11):1797–803.

99. Grassetto G, Marzola MC, Minicozzi A, et al. F-18 FDG PET/CT in rectal carcinoma: where are we now? Clin Nucl Med 2011;36:884–8.

100. Muthusamy VR, Chang KJ. Optimal methods for staging rectal cancer. Clin Cancer Res 2007;13:6877S–84S.

101. Curvo-Semedo L, Lambregts DM, Maas M, et al. Diffusion-weighted MRI in rectal cancer: apparent diffusion coefficient as a potential noninvasive marker of tumor aggressiveness. J Magn Reson Imaging 2012;35(6):1365–71.

102. Lambregts DM, Cappendijk VC, Maas M, et al. Value of MRI and diffusion-weighted MRI for the diagnosis of locally recurrent rectal cancer. Eur Radiol 2011;21:1250–8.

103. Denecke T, Rau B, Hoffmann KT, et al. Comparison of CT, MRI and FDG-PET in response prediction of patients with locally advanced rectal cancer after multimodal preoperative therapy: is there a benefit in using functional imaging? Eur Radiol 2005;15(8):1658–66.

104. Schmidt GP, Baur-Melnyk A, Haug A, et al. Whole-body MRI at 1.5 T and 3 T compared with FDG-PET-CT for the detection of tumour recurrence in patients with colorectal cancer. Eur Radiol 2009;19(6):1366–78.

105. Maegerlein C, Fingerle AA, Souvatzoglou M, et al. Detection of liver metastases in patients with adenocarcinomas of the gastrointestinal tract: comparison of (18)F-FDG PET/CT and MR imaging. Abdom Imaging 2015;40(5):1213–22.

106. Paspulati RM, Partovi S, Herrmann KA, et al. Comparison of hybrid FDG PET/MRI compared with PET/CT in colorectal cancer staging and restaging: a pilot study. Abdom Imaging 2015;40(6):1415–25.

107. Sassen S, de Booij M, Sosef M, et al. Locally advanced rectal cancer: is diffusion weighted MRI helpful for the identification of complete responders (ypT0N0) after neoadjuvant chemoradiation therapy? Eur Radiol 2013;23(12):3440–9.

108. Joye I, Deroose CM, Vandecaveye V, et al. The role of diffusion-weighted MRI and (18)F-FDG PET/CT in the prediction of pathologic complete response after radiochemotherapy for rectal cancer: a systematic review. Radiother Oncol 2014;113(2):158–65.

109. Song I, Kim SH, Lee SJ, et al. Value of diffusion-weighted imaging in the detection of viable tumour after neoadjuvant chemoradiation therapy in patients with locally advanced rectal cancer: comparison with T2 weighted and PET/CT imaging. Br J Radiol 2012;85(1013):577–86.

110. Iagaru A, Quon A, McDougall IR, et al. F-18 FDG PET/CT evaluation of osseous and soft tissue sarcomas. Clin Nucl Med 2006 Dec;31(12):754–60.

111. Rauscher I, Eiber M, Fürst S, et al. PET/MR imaging in the detection and characterization of pulmonary lesions: technical and diagnostic evaluation in comparison to PET/CT. J Nucl Med 2014;55(5):724–9.

The Emerging Role of PET/MR Imaging in Gynecologic Cancers

Maria Rosana Ponisio, MD[a], Kathryn J. Fowler, MD[b,c],
Farrokh Dehdashti, MD[a,c],*

KEYWORDS

- PET/MR imaging • Gynecologic malignancies • Uterine cervical cancer
- Uterine endometrial cancer • Ovarian epithelial cancer

KEY POINTS

- PET with 2-deoxy-2-[18F]-fluoro-D-glucose (FDG) has a role in staging gynecologic malignancies.
- Current data show that PET/computed tomography (CT) and PET/MR imaging have similar diagnostic performance for detection of malignant lesions with the advantage of significant reductions in radiation exposure by removing the CT component of PET/CT, which is especially important in this population undergoing serial examinations.
- FDG-PET/MR imaging may improve the diagnostic accuracy for local and distant metastatic disease because of the superior soft tissue contrast of MR imaging compared with CT.
- Functional MR techniques and multiparametric imaging applications such as diffusion-weighted imaging and dynamic contrast-enhanced imaging improve the characterization of lesions and provide quantitative biomarkers for assessment of response to treatment.
- Patients with gynecologic malignancies who require both PET and MR imaging should undergo a simultaneous PET/MR imaging examination that combines metabolic, anatomic, and functional imaging and decreases misregistration caused by patient motion or physiologic changes/motion of various organs.

INTRODUCTION

This article summarizes the current literature on PET/MR imaging in gynecologic malignancies and outlines the emerging clinical value of PET/MR imaging as an imaging tool in the management of the 3 most common gynecologic cancers: uterine cervical, uterine endometrial, and ovarian epithelial. Our experience with simultaneous PET/MR imaging is used to show the advantages and challenges of this new hybrid imaging modality in patients with gynecologic cancers.

In the last decades, the standard of care for the initial staging and the subsequent assessment of treatment response for many cancers has become PET in conjunction with computed tomography (CT) using the glucose analogue 2-deoxy-2-[18F]-fluoro-D-glucose (FDG).[1–3] Despite its central role, FDG-PET/CT has well-recognized limitations with respect to local tumor staging and the characterization of certain lesions in patients with gynecologic cancer.[4] In these cases, because imaging is central to staging as well as determining

Disclosure: The authors have nothing to disclose.
[a] Division of Nuclear Medicine, Edward Mallinckrodt Institute of Radiology, Washington University School of Medicine, 510 South Kingshighway Boulevard, St Louis, MO 63110, USA; [b] Division of Abdominal Imaging, Edward Mallinckrodt Institute of Radiology, Washington University School of Medicine, 510 South Kingshighway Boulevard, St Louis, MO 63110, USA; [c] Alvin J. Siteman Cancer Center, Washington University School of Medicine, 510 South Kingshighway Boulevard, St Louis, MO 63110, USA
* Corresponding author.
E-mail address: dehdashtif@wustl.edu

PET Clin 11 (2016) 425–440
http://dx.doi.org/10.1016/j.cpet.2016.05.005

prognosis and treatment strategy, further evaluation with MR imaging can be performed to ensure proper clinical management. The role of MR imaging is well established in gynecologic cancers, because it complements the molecular and metabolic data of PET with its superior soft tissue contrast and anatomic resolution, lack of ionizing radiation, and the ability to assess cellular density by MR based diffusion weighted imaging (DWI) and tissue perfusion and oxygenation by dynamic contrast-enhanced (DCE) MR imaging.[5–7] Accordingly, PET/MR imaging has significant potential to positively affect patient care by improving the diagnosis, initial staging, and subsequent management decisions in patients with gynecologic cancers.

Over the last few years, the increased number of PET/MR imaging installations in clinical settings and the growing evidence with respect to its utility have provided a deeper understanding of the benefits of the routine clinical use of PET/MR imaging to justify the added expense and complexity compared with PET/CT. This article summarizes the current body of evidence on gynecologic cancers, and delineates the limitations of these two hybrid imaging modalities as related to current challenges and areas likely to benefit from the clinical use of PET/MR imaging. It presents case examples to show the specific advantages of simultaneous PET/MR imaging based on our experience with gynecologic cancers in a clinical setting.

PET/MR IMAGING TECHNICAL BACKGROUND

In order to better understand the inherent advantages, disadvantages, and limitations of PET/MR imaging, this article briefly discusses their design and development. At present, PET/MR imaging systems can acquire MR and PET data either simultaneously or sequentially. Integrated PET/MR imaging systems simultaneously acquire PET and MR imaging data allowing concurrent imaging of the same region within a single gantry housing both the MR imaging and PET scanners. In the sequential PET/MR imaging acquisition, spatially separate individual PET and MR imaging scanners are connected by a common moving table that functions to reduce changes in patient positioning between imaging examinations. The installed base of PET/MR imaging systems currently comprises approximately 80% simultaneous acquisition units, driven by the multimodality multiparametric imaging capabilities in both the spatial and temporal domains of this hybrid modality.[8]

At present, the most critical limitation of both sequential and simultaneous PET/MR imaging

examinations is the accuracy of the MR imaging-derived attenuation correction (MR-AC) algorithms for PET. In PET/CT, the CT-derived attenuation correction is directly generated from the electron density information yielding photon-corrected PET images. Unlike CT, the MR imaging signal acquired during PET/MR imaging instead correlates with proton density and tissue relaxation properties and does not reflect electron density. Thus, alternate attenuation correction methods were developed for PET/MR imaging. The current approaches to MR-AC can be classified into 3 categories: segmentation, atlas, and emissions-based methods.[9–12] In the clinical whole-body imaging setting, MR-AC is typically derived from a segmentation-based method using Dixon sequences followed by image segmentation that classifies voxels into 4 classes of tissues (eg, background/air, soft tissue, fat, lung), creating an attenuation map. This approach uses the patient's imaging data and thus is reasonably accurate to account for anatomic and physiologic variants. Although there have been steady improvements in segmentation-based MR-AC methodologies, many technical problems remain. Correct delineation of the lung parenchyma may occasionally fail; Dixon classifications may generate incorrect voxel tissue values; and patient motion, both physiologic and nonphysiologic, all can result in artifacts that propagate into the MR-AC PET images and thus affect clinical image interpretation.[13] In addition, current segmentation-based MR attenuation maps are derived without cortical bone being included because cortical bone does not provide adequate MR imaging signal to be represented in MR-AC maps. Thus, the standard Dixon method does not account for cortical bone, resulting in local underestimation of standardized uptake values (SUVs) for tissues adjacent to or within cortical bone compared with PET/CT.[14] Although these limitations exist, the current MR-AC methods are likely sufficient for clinical use (ie, when highly precise SUV measurements are not necessary to diagnose and follow treatment response for most lesions).

PET/MR IMAGING PROTOCOL AND WORK-FLOW DESIGN

At the authors' institution, PET/MR imaging examinations are performed on a simultaneous 3T PET/MR imaging system (Siemens Biograph mMR; Siemens Health Care, Erlangen, Germany). The whole-body PET/MR imaging protocol is complemented by dedicated pelvis sequences in patients with gynecologic cancers. The MR imaging provides different image contrasts through adjustments of echo and repetition times, parameters that represent specific tissue characteristics. T1-weighted and T2-weighted sequences are the foundation of morphologic imaging, and these high-resolution sequences are acquired simultaneously with PET data. High-resolution T2-weighted images provide details of the uterine and cervical zonal anatomy and external contours, assisting in assessment of parametrial invasion. The isotropic three-dimensional (3D) T2-weighted fast (turbo) spin echo imaging sequence (in Siemens' nomenclature Sampling Perfection with Application optimized Contrasts using different flip angle Evolution [SPACE]), which optimizes contrast using flip angle evolution and allows for reformation of images in the axial, sagittal, and coronal planes without loss of resolution, and thus decreases the duration of the examination. DWI and the quantitative apparent diffusion coefficient (ADC) maps contribute to tumor delineation and characterization, and evaluation of therapy response. Administration of gadolinium-based intravenous contrast material helps to better characterize invasion of local structures and assessment of other pelvic structures (eg, lymph nodes and ovaries). PET acquisition is typically performed over 3 to 5 bed positions to cover the skull base to upper thighs with an acquisition time of 2 to 3 minutes per bed position, resulting in a total study time of approximately 20 minutes. **Table 1** lists the nominal sequence parameters used at the authors' institution.

GYNECOLOGIC CANCERS

One of the most significant worldwide public health issues and a leading cause of morbidity and mortality in women of all ages is gynecologic cancer. The classification of gynecologic cancers is based on the anatomic origin of the primary site, with the most common cancers being uterine cervical, uterine endometrial, and ovarian epithelial. In the United States alone, an estimated 105,890 women will be diagnosed with gynecologic cancers and 30,890 women will die of these cancers in 2016.[46] Most gynecologic cancers are staged clinically using the International Federation of Gynecology and Obstetrics (FIGO) criteria. The use of imaging has been shown to greatly benefit the care of the general oncology population, with FDG-PET/CT having a key role in the diagnosis, staging, and treatment monitoring/assessing.[15–18] In gynecologic cancers, the large variance with regard to location, staging, and prognosis has made imaging essential to the management of these patients. PET/CT provides functional and anatomic information with limited tissue contrast, whereas MR imaging provides better soft tissue resolution and contrast. Thus, the emerging new hybrid imaging modality of PET/MR imaging has the potential to expand the range of options available for detection, staging, treatment planning, and treatment response in gynecologic cancers. Evaluation of PET/MR imaging in gynecologic oncology has been performed by several groups.[19,20] Most of the current publications are based on small sample sizes, but preliminary results indicate that PET/MR imaging may perform better than PET/CT with respect to local tumor/node/metastasis (TNM) staging.

THE POTENTIAL ADDED VALUE OF ADVANCED MR IMAGING TECHNIQUES IN GYNECOLOGIC CANCERS

The rapid advances in MR imaging technology in terms of increased field strength (3T), development of new imaging techniques to shorten acquisition times (parallel imaging), and new functional sequences, which provide better characterization of tumors, have led to improvements in MR imaging for gynecologic cancers.

At present, MR imaging has an essential and well-established role in the management of patients with cervical and ovarian cancer, and a promising role in patients with endometrial carcinoma. The specific benefits are addressed later for each disease process individually. The superior soft tissue contrast, resolution, and multiplanar capabilities of MR imaging allow accurate determination of tumor location, tumor size, extension, and nodal involvement. It is now routinely used in staging, treatment monitoring, and detection of recurrent disease.

Beyond anatomic delineation of tumor, the potential of functional MR imaging lies in its ability to overcome the limitations of conventional MR imaging by providing biological information about the tumor to better distinguish between posttreatment changes and residual or recurrent disease. The clinical application of functional MR imaging in gynecologic cancers focuses on DCE MR imaging and DWI, which provide biological information related to tumor oxygenation, perfusion, and microstructure. In addition, functional MR imaging–derived quantitative parameters can potentially act as biomarkers for response assessment.[21–23] In **Table 2**, publications on the utility of DCE MR imaging and DWI for the 3 most common gynecologic cancers are presented.[19,24,25]

DCE MR imaging is a dynamic imaging technique that quantifies the pharmacokinetic profile of an injected intravenous bolus of gadolinium-based

Table 1
PET/MR imaging sequence parameters

Sequence Parameters	T1-weighted Precontrast and Postcontrast Fat-suppressed Images	Diffusion-weighted Images	Isotropic 3D T2-weighted (SPACE) Images	T2-weighted High-resolution TSE Images	2-Point Dixon Images	FDG-PET Images
Whole Body						
Acquisition time	18–20 s	3–4 min	—	—	18–20 s/station (simultaneous with PET)	90 s/station (4–5 stations from skull vertex to thighs)
Slice thickness	3–5 mm	5 mm	—	—	4 mm	—
b values (mm²/s)	—	At least 1000	—	—	—	—
Pelvis						
Acquisition time	18–20 s	5–7 min	6–9 min	7–9 min	18–20 s/station (simultaneous with PET)	90 s/station (4–5 stations from skull vertex to thighs)
Slice thickness	3–5 mm	3–5 mm	2–3 mm	3 mm (orthogonal to cervix)	4 mm	—
b values (mm²/s)	—	At least 1000	—	—	—	—
Clinical application	Assist in tumor localization and extension	DWI and ADC map assess tumor cellularity	Evaluation for myometrial and parametrial invasion A potential substitute for multiplanar T2-weighted images	Evaluation of myometrial and parametrial invasion	MR imaging–based segmentation	Metabolic information

Table 2
Role of DCE MR imaging and DWI in gynecologic cancers

Study, Year	Number of Patients	Primary Cancer	Findings
Brandmaier et al,[24] 2015	31	Cervical cancer	Significant inverse correlation between SUV_{max} and ADC_{min} in primary tumors and recurrent local tumors ($P<.05$)
Grueneisen et al,[19] 2014	14	Cervical cancer	Strong inverse correlation between SUV_{max} and ADC_{min} of primary lesions ($P<.001$), although recurrent lesions did not show a significant correlation
Shih et al,[25] 2015	47	Endometrial cancer	SUV_{max} and ADC_{min} are inversely correlated and are associated with pathologic prognostic factors ($P<.05$)

Abbreviations: ADC_{min}, minimum ADC; SUV_{max}, maximum SUV.

contrast agent before, during, and after its administration to assess tissue perfusion and oxygenation. The signal intensity changes in the images allow the derivation of a dynamic time–signal intensity curve in a region of interest, generating parametric maps of specific tumor microvasculature biomarkers.

DWI measures the molecular diffusion of water within voxels, providing an approximation of tissue cellularity and membrane integrity during the MR imaging pulse sequence. Determining the difference in the diffusion of water molecules allows for the characterization of the tissue because impeded diffusion (increased cellularity) is associated with lesions, whereas normal background tissues generally have greater diffusion (decreased cellularity). The signal intensity seen on DWI is a function of the sensitizing diffusion gradient, b value, which is proportional to the gradient amplitude. As the b values are increased, the signal intensity associated with tissue cellularity changes (becomes more bright) and the signal intensities of selected tissues, such as bowel or background fat, are suppressed for the purpose of better lesion detection. Quantitative analysis of DWI may be performed with the ADC maps derived from the exponential attenuation of signal intensity between diffusion images obtained at 2 or more different b values. The ADC maps assess changes in cellularity over time, providing a quantitative biomarker for response to treatment.

THE ROLE OF PET/MR IMAGING IN GYNECOLOGIC CANCERS
Uterine Cervical Cancer

Staging
Uterine cervical cancer is the fourth most commonly diagnosed cancer, with an estimated

527,600 new cases, and was the fourth leading cause of cancer deaths in women worldwide in 2012 with an estimated 265,700 deaths.[26] Nearly 90% of cervical cancer deaths occurred in developing countries, mainly because of a lack of screening to detect and remove precancerous lesions.[27,28] Most cervical cancers are caused by persistent infection of the cervical epithelium by one of the oncogenic human papilloma virus types. On histology, squamous cell carcinomas account for approximately 80% of all cervical cancers, adenocarcinoma accounts for approximately 15%, and the remainder comprise rarer histologic types such as adenoma malignum, adenosquamous carcinoma, neuroendocrine tumor, small cell tumor, and rhabdomyosarcoma.

Cervical cancer has a predictable dissemination, with initial invasion of local structures and regional lymph nodes, and later hematogenous spread to distant organs. Tumors spread locally to the lower uterine segment, vagina, and paracervical space; invade neighboring organs such as the rectum and bladder; and extend to the sidewalls of the pelvis. The dissemination to the lymph nodes outside the local area follows a sequential pattern, from pelvic lymph nodes to para-aortic nodes to supraclavicular nodes.

Since 2009, a revised FIGO staging system has been used for cervical cancer[29] (**Table 3**). The FIGO staging system is based on clinical evaluation with the procedures limited to physical examination, colposcopy, biopsy, conization of the cervix, cystoscopy, and proctosigmoidoscopy. A major limitation of FIGO staging is the lack of consideration of locoregional nodal involvement and the lack of use of the results of advanced imaging modalities (CT, MR imaging, and PET) in determining disease stage. This limitation has resulted in staging and treatment monitoring using

Table 3
FIGO staging of cervical cancer

Stage I	Tumor limited to the uterine cervix
IA1	Tumor confined to the cervix, diagnosed only by microscopy with invasion of ≤3 mm in depth and lateral spread ≤7 mm
IA2	Confined to the cervix, diagnosed with microscopy with invasion of >3 mm and ≤5 mm with lateral spread ≤7 mm
IB1	Clinically visible lesion or microscopic lesion greater than IA2, ≤4 cm in greatest dimension
IB2	Clinically visible lesion, >4 cm in greatest dimension
Stage II	Cervical carcinoma invades beyond uterus but not to pelvic wall or to lower third of vagina
IIA1	Involvement of the upper two-thirds of the vagina, without parametrial invasion, ≤4 cm in greatest dimension
IIA2	Involvement of the upper two-thirds of the vagina, without parametrial invasion, >4 cm in greatest dimension
IIB	With parametrial invasion
Stage III	Tumor extends to pelvic wall and/or involves lower third of vagina and/or causes hydronephrosis or nonfunctional kidney
IIIA	Tumor involves lower third of vagina, no extension to pelvic wall
IIIB	Tumor extends to pelvic wall and/or causes hydronephrosis or nonfunctional kidney
Stage IV	Tumor invades mucosa of bladder or rectum and/or extends beyond true pelvis
IVA	Tumor invasion of bladder or rectum
IVB	Tumor extends beyond true pelvis

From Pecorelli S. Revised FIGO staging for carcinoma of the vulva, cervix, and endometrium. Int J Gynaecol Obstet 2009;105:103–4; with permission. © 2009 by the International Federation of Gynecology and Obstetrics.

surgical and histopathologic staging classifications (TNM and Union for International Cancer Control [UICC]).

Treatment is linked to disease stage and imaging plays an important role in determining appropriate management. The treatment of early-stage cervical cancer is surgery or definitive radiation therapy. In patients with FIGO stages I and IIA1, the typical treatment is surgery, and, in selected patients with lesions that are less than or equal to 2 cm in diameter, radical trachelectomy and laparoscopic pelvic lymphadenectomy can provide a fertility-sparing option. In patients with FIGO stage IB2 or higher, radiation therapy with concurrent chemotherapy is recommended. Treatment planning and options for cervical cancer have expanded, in part because of advances in imaging, although imaging does not modify the FIGO staging classifications. The current National Comprehensive Cancer Network (NCCN) guidelines recommend radiologic imaging (CT, PET/CT, and MR imaging) as indicated for stage IB2 or higher and as optional for stage IB1 or lower. In addition, the guidelines recommend imaging to determine distant metastases and tumor recurrences, and describe specific imaging modality

application pairing (1) CT-based treatment planning for external beam radiotherapy, (2) MR imaging for determining soft tissue and parametrial involvement, and (3) PET for defining nodal involvement.

In clinical practice, FDG-PET is increasingly used as an alternative to surgical lymph node dissection and in the evaluation of tumor volume, which also provides information on patient prognosis.[30] In addition, FDG-PET can assist in image-guided intensity modulated radiation therapy (IMRT). IMRT allows the use of higher radiation doses than traditional therapies and spares more of the surrounding healthy tissues.

The NCCN practice guidelines for cervical cancer[31,32] recognize the central role for imaging, because it significantly affects the detection, treatment planning, and assessment of treatment response. Although not included in FIGO staging classification, involvement of lymph nodes is correlated with the worst patient outcome. The role of PET in cervical cancer[33,34] is well documented and established. Most cervical cancers show increased FDG uptake, measured by the maximum SUV (SUV_{max}). In addition to semiquantitative information about the patient's primary tumor, which helps to define the tumor volume and predict prognosis, accurate evaluation of involvement of adjacent structures (parametrium, rectum, and bladder) represents an important determinant for the selection of appropriate treatment. Multiple studies have shown PET/MR imaging to have high diagnostic image quality for the assessment of primary tumor and tumor infiltration into adjacent soft tissues (**Fig. 1**). In the literature, several studies have shown the diagnostic value of integrated PET/MR imaging for staging cervical cancer in pretreated patients. Representative of these studies, the work by Grueneisen and colleagues[35] showed that PET/MR imaging detected all cervical lesions in 27 patients, allowing the correct determination of the T stage in 85% of cases, and had sensitivity, specificity, and diagnostic accuracy of 91%, 94%, and 93%, respectively, for detection of lymph node metastasis. High-resolution T2-weighted imaging is best for depicting the cervical

stromal and parametrial invasion, with multiplanar T2-weighted imaging serving as the standard approach. Newer-generation sequences, such as isotropic 3D T2-weighted (SPACE) imaging may allow high-quality multiplanar images to be obtained following a single acquisition, in which isotropic voxels can be reconstructed in multiple planes without significant loss of resolution (**Fig. 2**).[36]

In patients with more advanced disease, FDG-PET has superior ability to detect regional and distant metastatic disease compared with CT and MR imaging alone (**Fig. 3**).[37,38] FDG uptake improves specificity and sensitivity of nodal metastatic determination compared with CT and MR imaging, because detection of lymph nodes metastasis is based on radiotracer uptake and not on standard size criteria morphologically. A meta-analysis of 41 studies[39] that compared the diagnostic performances of CT, MR imaging, and

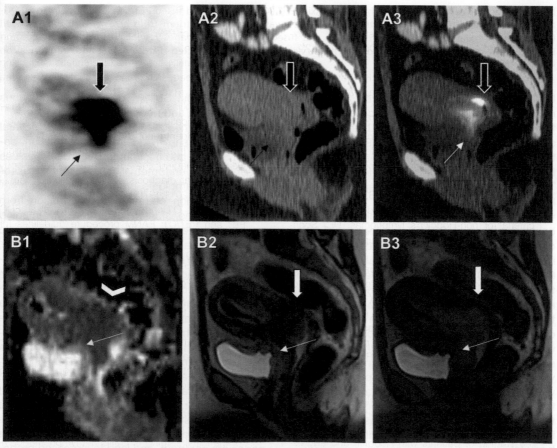

Fig. 1. Squamous cell carcinoma of the cervix. Sagittal PET (*A1*), CT (*A2*), and fused PET/CT (*A3*) images show FDG-avid cervical mass involving uterus and upper vagina (*thick arrows*) with questionable invasion of bladder wall (*thin arrows*). Sagittal ADC map (*B1*), isotropic 3D T2-weighted (SPACE) MR (*B2*), and fused PET/MR (*B3*) images provide better soft tissue resolution showing direct extension into bladder trigone (*thin arrows*). The cervical mass shows restricted diffusion on ADC map images (*B1, arrowhead*).

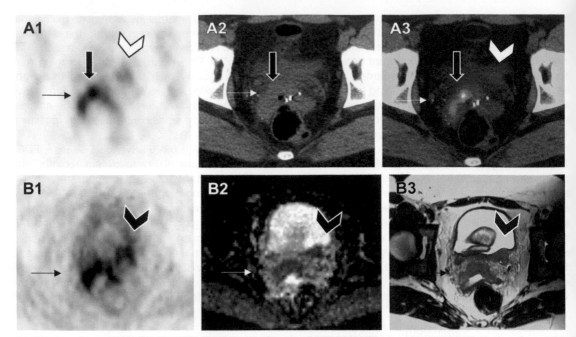

Fig. 2. Squamous cell carcinoma of the cervix. Axial PET (*A1*), CT (*A2*), and fused PET/CT (*A3*) images show FDG-avid cervical mass (*thick arrows*) with questionable invasion of parametrium (*thin arrows*) and bladder wall (*arrowheads*). Axial PET (*B1*), ADC map (*B2*), and fused PET/MR (*B3*) images reveal FDG-avid tumor bulging into adjacent parametrium (*thin arrows*). The cervical mass shows restricted diffusion (*B2*) and frank invasion into posterior bladder (*arrowheads*).

PET or PET/CT for detection of metastatic lymph nodes in patients with cervical cancer showed that PET or PET/CT showed the highest pooled sensitivity (82%) and specificity (95%), whereas those of CT were 50% and 92%, and those of MR imaging were 56% and 91%, respectively. The retrospective study by Kitajima and colleagues[40] showed that software fusion of PET with MR imaging had comparable results with contrast-enhanced PET/CT for the identification of lymph node metastases with a sensitivity, specificity, and accuracy for both modalities of 92.3%, 88.2%, and 90.0%, respectively. New MR imaging techniques may further enhance detection of nodal and distant metastases. The improved soft tissue contrast of MR imaging compared with CT can help distinguish normal anatomic structures with physiologic uptake from pathologic uptake such as differentiating between normal ovaries versus metastatic lymph nodes in premenopausal women. Likewise, the improved spatial coregistration can alleviate confusion related to bowel uptake that may also masquerade as nodal uptake in the pelvis of patients with minimal intrinsic body fat.

Prognosis/prediction

The SUV_{max} of primary tumors varies, based on the histology and degree of tumor differentiation, with the highest SUV_{max} observed in squamous cell carcinoma and poorly differentiated tumors.[41] Using simultaneous PET/MR imaging, several studies have shown an inverse correlation between SUV_{max} and minimum ADC (ADC_{min}) values in cervical and endometrial cancers that are associated with pathologic prognostic factors.[24,35,42] The combination of metabolic information from PET and functional information from MR imaging may provide complementary prognostic biomarker data in gynecologic cancers.

Lymph node involvement, in addition to determination of management, has been shown to provide prognostic and predictive information. Patients with PET-positive lymph nodes have significantly worse survival rates than those with PET-negative lymph nodes. The disease-specific survival rates can be stratified into distinct groups based on the most distant level of FDG-PET positive nodal disease, the groups being none; pelvic; pelvic and para-aortic; or pelvic, para-aortic, and supraclavicular.[41,43] In cases of advance cervical cancer (FIGO stages III and IVA), distant metastases in the para-aortic and supraclavicular lymph nodes are common, and lead to increased probability of tumor recurrence and lower survival rates. Most patients with advanced stage cervical cancer develop recurrence within 2 years after initial treatment, with approximately 70% of the patients

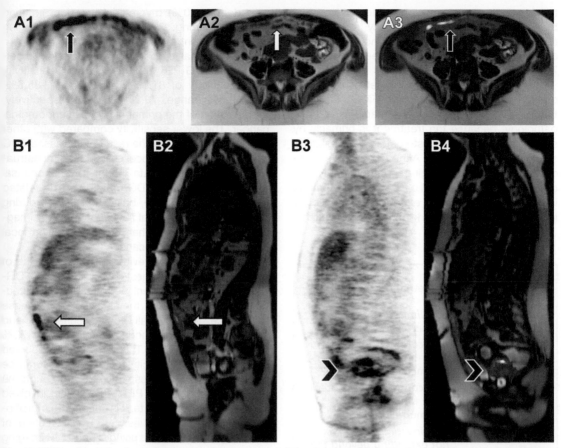

Fig. 3. FIGO stage IVB adenocarcinoma of the cervix. Axial PET (*A1*), T2-weighted MR (*A2*), fused T2-weighted MR/PET (*A3*), sagittal PET (*B1*), and sagittal fused T2-weighted MR/PET (*B2*) images show hypermetabolic omental nodularity (*arrows*), in keeping with peritoneal carcinomatosis, correlating with biopsy-proven results. Sagittal PET (*B3*) and sagittal fused T2-weighted MR/PET (*B4*) images show FDG-avid primary cervical mass (*arrowheads*).

surviving the recurrence. Thus, early disease detection when the disease can be treated effectively is the key to increased survival rates, and multiple studies have shown that FDG-PET is pivotal for this role. In a recent meta-analysis, the derived pooled sensitivity and specificity was 91% (95% confidence interval [CI], 87%–94%) and 94% (95% CI, 89%–97%) for PET, respectively, and 92% (95% CI, 91%–94%) and 84% (95% CI, 74%–91%) for PET/CT, respectively.[44] Published studies with small numbers of patients have shown that the diagnostic accuracy of PET/MR imaging is similar to that of PET/CT. In one study of 19 patients with recurrent cervical cancer, PET/MR imaging showed similar diagnostic accuracy to PET/CT, identifying all local and distant recurrent disease sites and providing greater interpretation confidence than PET/CT ($P<.001$).[45]

Clinical assessment of response to treatment can be challenging because most patients continue with previous symptoms such as pain and discharge. Moreover, physical examination does not necessarily reflect the presence of active disease. Multiple studies have shown that FDG-PET findings after primary therapy are the most significant predictive factors for tumor recurrence and life expectancy of cervical cancer compared with pretreatment and treatment-related prognostic factors.[46,47]

Endometrial Cancer

Endometrial cancer is the most frequent gynecologic cancer occurring in Western countries. In the United States, for 2016, an estimated 60,050 new cases of endometrial cancer are expected to be diagnosed, and 10,470 women will die of this cancer.[48] In less developed nations, endometrial cancer is rare because risk factors like obesity and excessive fat consumption are much less common. There is no routine screening test for this cancer, and thus most cases are diagnosed because of abnormal uterine bleeding, with diagnostic assessment performed by transvaginal ultrasonography and endometrial biopsy. The diagnosis is usually made early, resulting in high survival rates, including 5-year and 10-year relative survival rates of 82% and 79%, respectively.

The formal staging of endometrial cancer is defined using the 2010 revised FIGO classification[29,49] (**Table 4**), from surgical staging and histopathology, because the treatment is primarily by surgery, consisting of hysterectomy and bilateral salpingo-oophorectomy. Although FIGO staging does not have an imaging component, NCCN guidelines for endometrial cancer[50,51] recommend imaging for evaluation of extrauterine disease, as indicated by clinical work-up. Thus, in patients with deep (>50%) myometrial invasion, imaging (CT, MR imaging, PET) is used for initial staging and assessment of treatment response.[52,53]

In a meta-analysis performed by Kakhki and colleagues,[54] FDG-PET and PET/CT had a sensitivity and specificity of 81.8% (range, 77.9%–85.3%) and 89.8% (range, 79.2%–96.2%), respectively for detection of the primary lesions in endometrial cancer. The lower sensitivity compared with other cancers is most likely the result of increased FDG uptake from benign processes such as menstruation and leiomyomata.[55] In premenopausal women, endometrial FDG uptake can be related to the menstrual cycle, being the highest during ovulatory and menstrual flow phases.[56] MR imaging is more accurate than CT in evaluating local staging in endometrial cancer.[57]

A recent systematic review and meta-analysis of the literature (31 studies) concluded that FDG-PET/CT has an excellent performance for detection of lymph node metastasis and disease recurrence. The overall pooled sensitivity and specificity for lymph node detection were 72% and 94%, respectively. The corresponding pooled sensitivity and specificity for disease recurrence were 95% and 91%, respectively.[58] Although the reported sensitivity for PET/CT to detect involved lymph nodes is moderate, it is superior to morphologic imaging techniques.[22,59] The detection of pathologic lymph nodes using CT and MR imaging is based on the short-axis nodal size, with diameters of greater than 10 mm being the most accepted criterion for the diagnosis of a node suspected to contain metastatic deposits. This criterion has low sensitivity and specificity.[60,61] The cause of the moderate sensitivity may be related to the spatial resolution of PET/CT for detection of metastatic lymph nodes in uterine cancer, given the reported sensitivity based on nodal size of 17% for lymph nodes less than 4 mm and 93% for lymph nodes greater than 10 mm.[62] The reported high negative predictive value (NPV) in presurgical evaluation with FDG-PET/CT may help to identify patients who will benefit from lymphadenectomy and, thus, decrease the morbidity associated with surgical complications.[63]

In terms of surveillance, a meta-analysis of the published literature showed that FDG-PET had pooled sensitivity and specificity of 28.7% and 35.4%, respectively, for detection of recurrent endometrial cancer, and was highly accurate in detection of local and distant recurrence. However, it was noted that the location of the site of recurrence may affect the performance of the FDG-PET.[64] FDG-PET was highly accurate in detection of local and distant recurrences, although its accuracy was higher for detection of

Table 4 FIGO staging of endometrial cancer	
Stage I	Tumor limited to the uterine corpus
IA	Tumor confined to the uterus, no or less than half of myometrial invasion
IB	Tumor confined to the uterus, more than half of myometrial invasion
Stage II	Tumor invading the cervix but not extending beyond the uterus
Stage III	Local or regional spread of tumor
IIIA	Tumor invades the serosa of the corpus uteri and/or adnexa
IIIB	Vaginal or parametrial involvement
IIIC1	Metastases to pelvic lymph nodes
IIIC2	Metastases to para-aortic lymph nodes
Stage IV	Tumor invading bladder or bowel mucosa or both, or distant metastases
IVA	Tumor invasion of bladder mucosa and/or bowel mucosa
IVB	Distant metastasis including abdominal metastases and/or inguinal lymph nodes

Note that uterine sarcomas have a different FIGO staging system.

From Pecorelli S. Revised FIGO staging for carcinoma of the vulva, cervix, and endometrium. Int J Gynaecol Obstet 2009;105:103–4; with permission. © 2009 by the International Federation of Gynecology and Obstetrics.

pelvic lymph node recurrence than for para-aortic lymph node recurrence.

MR imaging plays an important role in assessing large masses and/or high-grade tumors (histologic grades 2 and 3), which have a high risk of extra-uterine dissemination (**Figs. 4** and **5**). MR imaging has high sensitivity (80%–85%)[65,66] and NPV (90%) for evaluation of myometrial invasion.[67] MR imaging is more accurate than CT and ultraso-nography in the identification of myometrial and cervical invasion. Contrast-enhanced T1-weighted images as well as T2-weighted images are of great utility for evaluation of myometrial,[68] cervical, and surrounding organ invasion.[69] A retrospective study showed a higher diagnostic performance of fused FDG-PET/MR imaging compared with FDG-PET/CT for evaluation of local, nodal, and distant recurrences in patients with gynecologic cancers.[70] In this study, patients underwent contrast-enhanced PET/CT and contrast-enhanced PET/MR imaging to evaluate their diag-nostic performances for assessment of the extent of recurrent disease. Overall, the performance of PET/MR imaging was superior to that of PET/CT. For example, fused PET/MR imaging and MR im-aging alone had an accuracy of 93.3%, whereas contrast-enhanced PET/CT had 80% accuracy for detection of local recurrences ($P<.041$).

One of the key strengths of the multimodality im-aging approach of PET/MR imaging is the avail-ability of multiparametric quantitative information. The study by Shih and colleagues[25] demonstrated the application of multiparametric maps by showing a significant inverse correlation between SUV$_{max}$ and ADC$_{min}$ of primary tumors in patients with endometrial cancer derived from simulta-neous PET/MR imaging, and their associations with pathologic prognostic factors. The 2 imaging biomarkers had strong associations, with SUV$_{max}$ being significantly higher in tumors with advanced stage, deep myometrial invasion, cervical inva-sion, lymphovascular space involvement, and lymph node metastasis, and ADC$_{min}$ being signifi-cantly lower in tumors with higher grade, advanced stage, and cervical invasion. In a study by Nakamura and colleagues,[23] ADC$_{min}$ of the primary tumor was the only independent prognos-ticator of disease recurrence ($P = .019$). Measure-ment of the ADC$_{min}$ of the primary tumor and serum cancer antigen 125 (CA-125) levels were predictive of disease recurrence for patients with endometrial cancer.

Ovarian Cancer

Ovarian cancer is the leading cause of death from gynecologic cancer in most Western nations, and is responsible for 5% of cancer deaths in women. In the United States, it is estimated that 22,280 new cases of ovarian cancer will be diagnosed and that 14,240 women will die of this disease in 2016.[48] The incidence of ovarian cancer increases with age, with most patients diagnosed in the postmenopausal period and presenting with advanced disease. Current routine screening is not recommended, and thus ovarian cancer is usually diagnosed based on patient history, tumor makers (typically CA-125), clinical palpation,

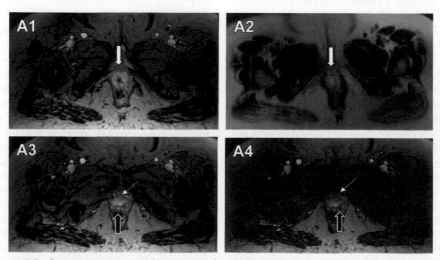

Fig. 4. Endometrial adenocarcinoma. Axial contrast-enhanced T1-weighted MR (*A1*, *A3*), fused T2-weighted MR/PET (*A2*), and fused contrast-enhanced T1-weighted MR/PET (*A4*) images show hypermetabolic circumferential enhancing nodules of distal vaginal wall (*thick white arrows*) with encasement of distal urethra (*thin arrows*) by soft tissue (*thick black arrows*), representing sites of tumor.

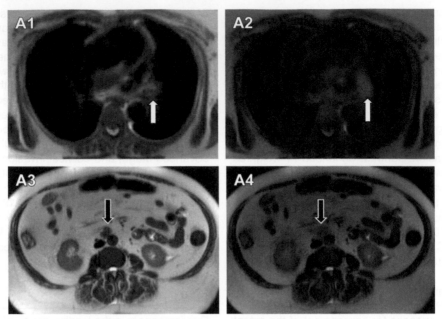

Fig. 5. Metastatic endometrial adenocarcinoma. Axial T2-weighted MR (*A1, A3*) and fused T2-weighted MR/PET (*A2, A4*) images show FDG-avid lymph nodes in left pulmonary hilum (*white arrows*) and retroperitoneum (*black arrows*), in keeping with metastatic disease.

and pelvic ultrasonography with histologic confirmation. Approximately 90% of ovarian cancers are epithelial carcinomas, including serous (the most common type), mucinous, endometrioid, clear cell, and undifferentiated subtypes.

The FIGO staging system is used for ovarian cancer, and is completely surgically based, defined by the extent and location of disease noted during cytoreduction (debulking) and biopsies. Tumor dissemination can occur in the peritoneal cavity through the parietal and visceral peritoneal layers, and through lymphatic pathways to involve inguinal, pelvic, para-aortic, suprarenal, mesenteric, mesocolic, and mediastinal lymph nodes. The most common extra-abdominal site of disease is the pleural space. The lack of clinical symptoms makes early detection of ovarian cancer challenging, and thus most patients present with disease of advanced stage (FIGO stages III–IV) at initial diagnosis. Exploratory laparotomy, cytoreduction, and chemotherapy are standard in the management of ovarian cancer.[71] However, intraoperative staging can underestimate the extent of disease, mainly because of unanticipated dissemination of disease, such as with spread to the abdominal peritoneal compartment and extrapelvic tumor deposits. Levels of the serum tumor marker, CA-125, are increased in more than 80% of patients with advanced disease, but increased levels can be encountered in the setting of benign lesions as well. Despite studies reporting

that this tumor marker is helpful to distinguish responder from nonresponder patients,[72] 10% of the patients have tumors classified as biomarker nonsecretors. The role of other serum tumor markers, such as human epididymis protein 4 (HE4), for improved detection of ovarian tumor is still not clear.[73]

The role of imaging is central in patient management and is fully addressed in the NCCN practice guidelines for ovarian cancer.[74–76] Clinically, imaging of the chest, abdomen, and pelvis via CT, MR imaging, or PET/CT is increasingly being used for preoperative evaluation of ovarian cancer to achieve complete tumor resection. Because residual tumor is an important prognostic factor, imaging may aid in determining the effectiveness of the surgery (**Fig. 6**). In addition, the combination of serum CA-125 testing and imaging now plays a pivotal role in assessing disease progression and response to therapy after surgical cytoreduction and adjuvant systemic therapy.

FDG-PET/CT has been shown to be superior to CT for staging and evaluation of disease preoperatively.[77] Furthermore, it has been reported that FDG-PET is a key determinant of patient outcome and recurrence risk,[20,78] and can identify metastatic lymph nodes with increased FDG uptake that are greater than 10 mm in size. The limited soft tissue resolution of CT may be overcome with the use of MR imaging, which allows more accurate detection of peritoneal involvement and better

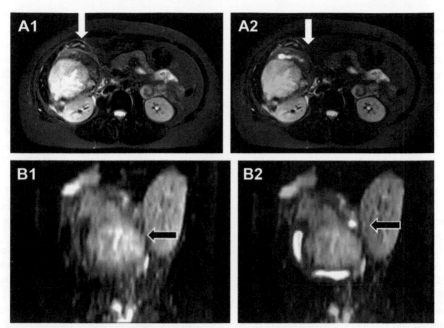

Fig. 6. Metastatic ovarian leiomyosarcoma. Axial fat-suppressed T2-weighted MR (*A1*), axial fused fat-suppressed T2-weighted MR/PET (*A2*), sagittal fat-suppressed T2-weighted MR (*B1*), and sagittal fused fat-suppressed T2-weighted MR/PET (*B2*) images show right upper quadrant peritoneal mass (*arrows*) with peripheral increased metabolic activity, representing residual metastatic tumor after cryoablation.

characterization of physiologic occasionally FDG-avid ovaries. Overall, MR imaging has been reported to be 95% sensitive and 82% specific for staging of ovarian cancer.[79] The detection of recurrent disease is challenging because of postoperative distortion of the complex pelvic anatomy. Several recent publications have shown the feasibility and high diagnostic value of whole-body simultaneous PET/MR imaging in patients with recurrent malignancy.[20,80,81] In a study by Beiderwellen and colleagues,[20] involving 19 patients with suspected recurrence of pelvic malignancy (ovarian cancer 11 patients, and cervical cancer 8 patients), PET/MR imaging not only had equivalent high diagnostic value for detection of recurrent disease on both a per-patient basis and a per-lesion basis compared with PET/CT but it also provided a higher diagnostic confidence in the discrimination of benign and malignant processes.

SUMMARY

Over the last few years, the increasing number of PET/MR imaging installations in clinical settings and the maturing body of evidence with respect to its utility has provided a deeper understanding of the benefits of routine clinical use of PET/MR imaging. Future research is needed to document improved outcomes and impact on patient

management relative to PET/CT. Despite the limited data regarding the role of whole-body FDG-PET/MR imaging in gynecologic cancers, preliminary experiences indicate that PET/MR imaging performance is equivalent to that of clinical PET/CT. Several studies have shown increased diagnostic confidence with PET/MR imaging based on its excellent soft tissue contrast and the application of functional techniques such as DWI and DCE MR imaging to better characterize lesions. Reduction in radiation exposure by removing the CT component of PET/CT is another advantage, especially in patient populations undergoing serial examinations. Some of the most promising aspects of PET/MR imaging are the emerging multimodality, multiparametric imaging applications, such as the derivation of SUV_{max} and ADC_{min} based on tumor metabolism and cellularity in gynecologic cancers. These two imaging biomarkers are associated with prognostic factors and may provide a better individual assessment of treatment response and of residual or recurrent disease.

Further studies in PET/MR imaging are needed to establish standardized acquisition protocols; to improve the implementations of MR-AC; and to develop new multimodality, multiparametric imaging techniques for producing and integrating the three types of imaging data: morphologic, functional, and molecular. Overall, the new hybrid imaging modality of PET/MR imaging will continue an evolution of adding diagnostic value compared with MR imaging and PET/CT alone, as new clinical applications emerge that add multimodality, multiparametric imaging.

REFERENCES

1. Brunetti J. PET/CT in gynecologic malignancies. Radiol Clin North Am 2013;51(5):895–911.
2. Delbeke D, Segall GM. Status of and trends in nuclear medicine in the United States. J Nucl Med 2011;52(Suppl 2):24S–8S.
3. Scheibler F, Zumbe P, Janssen I, et al. Randomized controlled trials on PET: a systematic review of topics, design, and quality. J Nucl Med 2012;53(7):1016–25.
4. Rockall AG, Cross S, Flanagan S, et al. The role of FDG-PET/CT in gynaecological cancers. Cancer Imaging 2012;12:49–65.
5. Namimoto T, Awai K, Nakaura T, et al. Role of diffusion-weighted imaging in the diagnosis of gynecological diseases. Eur Radiol 2009;19(3):745–60.
6. Ratner ES, Staib LH, Cross SN, et al. The clinical impact of gynecologic MRI. AJR Am J Roentgenol 2015;204(3):674–80.
7. Hameeduddin A, Sahdev A. Diffusion-weighted imaging and dynamic contrast-enhanced MRI in assessing response and recurrent disease in gynaecological malignancies. Cancer Imaging 2015;15:3.
8. Bailey DL, Pichler BJ, Guckel B, et al. Combined PET/MRI: multi-modality Multi-parametric imaging is here: summary report of the 4th International Workshop on PET/MR Imaging; February 23-27, 2015, Tubingen, Germany. Mol Imaging Biol 2015;17(5):595–608.
9. Mehranian A, Zaidi H. Clinical assessment of emission- and segmentation-based MR-guided attenuation correction in whole-body time-of-flight PET/MR imaging. J Nucl Med 2015;56(6):877–83.
10. Martinez-Moller A, Nekolla SG. Attenuation correction for PET/MR: problems, novel approaches and practical solutions. Z Med Phys 2012;22(4):299–310.
11. Eiber M, Martinez-Moller A, Souvatzoglou M, et al. Value of a Dixon-based MR/PET attenuation correction sequence for the localization and evaluation of PET-positive lesions. Eur J Nucl Med Mol Imaging 2011;38(9):1691–701.
12. Hofmann M, Bezrukov I, Mantlik F, et al. MRI-based attenuation correction for whole-body PET/MRI: quantitative evaluation of segmentation- and atlas-based methods. J Nucl Med 2011;52(9):1392–9.
13. Keller SH, Holm S, Hansen AE, et al. Image artifacts from MR-based attenuation correction in clinical, whole-body PET/MRI. MAGMA 2013;26(1):173–81.
14. Kim JH, Lee JS, Song IC, et al. Comparison of segmentation-based attenuation correction methods for PET/MRI: evaluation of bone and liver standardized uptake value with oncologic PET/CT data. J Nucl Med 2012;53(12):1878–82.
15. Zor E, Stokkel MP, Ozalp S, et al. F^{18}-FDG coincidence-PET in patients with suspected gynecological malignancy. Acta Radiol 2006;47(6):612–7.
16. Nishiyama Y, Yamamoto Y, Kanenishi K, et al. Monitoring the neoadjuvant therapy response in gynecological cancer patients using FDG PET. Eur J Nucl Med Mol Imaging 2008;35(2):287–95.
17. Amit A, Person O, Keidar Z. FDG PET/CT in monitoring response to treatment in gynecological malignancies. Curr Opin Obstet Gynecol 2013;25(1):17–22.
18. Bourguet P. Standards, Options and Recommendations for the use of PET-FDG in cancerology. Results in gynecological neoplasms. Bull Cancer 2003;90:S47–55 [in French].
19. Grueneisen J, Schaarschmidt BM, Beiderwellen K, et al. Diagnostic value of diffusion-weighted imaging in simultaneous ^{18}F-FDG PET/MR imaging for whole-body staging of women with pelvic malignancies. J Nucl Med 2014;55(12):1930–5.
20. Beiderwellen K, Grueneisen J, Ruhlmann V, et al. [(18)F]FDG PET/MRI vs. PET/CT for whole-body staging in patients with recurrent malignancies of the female pelvis: initial results. Eur J Nucl Med Mol Imaging 2015;42(1):56–65.
21. Harry VN. Novel imaging techniques as response biomarkers in cervical cancer. Gynecol Oncol 2010;116(2):253–61.
22. Salvesen HB, Haldorsen IS, Trovik J. Markers for individualised therapy in endometrial carcinoma. Lancet Oncol 2012;13(8):e353–361.
23. Nakamura K, Imafuku N, Nishida T, et al. Measurement of the minimum apparent diffusion coefficient (ADCmin) of the primary tumor and CA125 are predictive of disease recurrence for patients with endometrial cancer. Gynecol Oncol 2012;124(2):335–9.
24. Brandmaier P, Purz S, Bremicker K, et al. Simultaneous [18F]FDG-PET/MRI: correlation of apparent diffusion coefficient (ADC) and standardized uptake value (SUV) in primary and recurrent cervical cancer. PLoS One 2015;10(11):e0141684.
25. Shih IL, Yen RF, Chen CA, et al. Standardized uptake value and apparent diffusion coefficient of endometrial cancer evaluated with integrated whole-body PET/MR: correlation with pathological prognostic factors. J Magn Reson Imaging 2015;42(6):1723–32.
26. American Cancer Society. Global cancer facts & figures. 3rd edition. Atlanta (GA): American Cancer Society; 2015.
27. Sepulveda C, Prado R. Effective cervical cytology screening programmes in middle-income

countries: the Chilean experience. Cancer Detect Prev 2005;29(5):405–11.

28. Arbyn M, Cuzick J. International agreement to join forces in synthesizing evidence on new methods for cervical cancer prevention. Cancer Lett 2009; 278(1):1–2.

29. Pecorelli S. Revised FIGO staging for carcinoma of the vulva, cervix, and endometrium. Int J Gynaecol Obstet 2009;105(2):103–4.

30. Miller TR, Grigsby PW. Measurement of tumor volume by PET to evaluate prognosis in patients with advanced cervical cancer treated by radiation therapy. Int J Radiat Oncol Biol Phys 2002;53(2):353–9.

31. Koh W-J, Greer BE, Abu-Rustum NR, et al. Cervical cancer. J Natl Compr Canc Netw 2013;11:320–43.

32. Koh W-J, Greer BE, Abu-Rustum NR, et al. Cervical cancer, version 2.2015. J Natl Compr Canc Netw 2015;13:395–404.

33. Rose PG, Adler LP, Rodriguez M, et al. Positron emission tomography for evaluating para-aortic nodal metastasis in locally advanced cervical cancer before surgical staging: a surgicopathologic study. J Clin Oncol 1999;17(1):41–5.

34. Buchmann I, Reinhardt M, Elsner K, et al. 2-(Fluorine-18)fluoro-2-deoxy-D-glucose positron emission tomography in the detection and staging of malignant lymphoma. A bicenter trial. Cancer 2001; 91(5):889–99.

35. Grueneisen J, Schaarschmidt BM, Heubner M, et al. Integrated PET/MRI for whole-body staging of patients with primary cervical cancer: preliminary results. Eur J Nucl Med Mol Imaging 2015;42(12): 1814–24.

36. Fraum TJ, Fowler KJ, McConathy J, et al. PET/MRI for the body imager: abdominal and pelvic oncologic applications. Abdom Imaging 2015;40(6): 1387–404.

37. Belhocine T, Thille A, Fridman V, et al. Contribution of whole-body 18FDG PET imaging in the management of cervical cancer. Gynecol Oncol 2002;87(1): 90–7.

38. Havrilesky LJ, Kulasingam SL, Matchar DB, et al. FDG-PET for management of cervical and ovarian cancer. Gynecol Oncol 2005;97(1):183–91.

39. Choi HJ, Ju W, Myung SK, et al. Diagnostic performance of computer tomography, magnetic resonance imaging, and positron emission tomography or positron emission tomography/computer tomography for detection of metastatic lymph nodes in patients with cervical cancer: meta-analysis. Cancer Sci 2010;101(6):1471–9.

40. Kitajima K, Suenaga Y, Ueno Y, et al. Fusion of PET and MRI for staging of uterine cervical cancer: comparison with contrast-enhanced (18)F-FDG PET/CT and pelvic MRI. Clin Imaging 2014;38(4):464–9.

41. Kidd EA, Spencer CR, Huettner PC, et al. Cervical cancer histology and tumor differentiation affect 18F-fluorodeoxyglucose uptake. Cancer 2009; 115(15):3548–54.

42. Kuang F, Ren J, Zhong Q, et al. The value of apparent diffusion coefficient in the assessment of cervical cancer. Eur Radiol 2013;23(4):1050–8.

43. Grigsby PW, Siegel BA, Dehdashti F. Lymph node staging by positron emission tomography in patients with carcinoma of the cervix. J Clin Oncol 2001; 19(17):3745–9.

44. Ding XP, Feng L, Ma L. Diagnosis of recurrent uterine cervical cancer: PET versus PET/CT: a systematic review and meta-analysis. Arch Gynecol Obstet 2014;290(4):741–7.

45. Beiderwellen K, Geraldo L, Ruhlmann V, et al. Accuracy of [18F]FDG PET/MRI for the detection of liver metastases. PLoS One 2015;10(9):e0137285.

46. Grigsby PW, Siegel BA, Dehdashti F, et al. Posttherapy [18F] fluorodeoxyglucose positron emission tomography in carcinoma of the cervix: response and outcome. J Clin Oncol 2004;22(11):2167–71.

47. Schwarz JK, Siegel BA, Dehdashti F, et al. Association of posttherapy positron emission tomography with tumor response and survival in cervical carcinoma. JAMA 2007;298(19):2289–95.

48. American Cancer Society. Cancer facts & figures 2016. Atlanta (GA): American Cancer Society; 2016.

49. Lewin SN, Herzog TJ, Barrena Medel NI, et al. Comparative performance of the 2009 international Federation of gynecology and obstetrics' staging system for uterine corpus cancer. Obstet Gynecol 2010;116(5):1141–9.

50. Greer BE, Koh WJ, Abu-Rustum N, et al. Uterine neoplasms. Clinical practice guidelines in oncology. J Natl Compr Canc Netw 2009;7:498–531.

51. Koh WJ, Greer BE, Abu-Rustum NR, et al. Uterine neoplasms, version 1.2014. J Natl Compr Canc Netw 2014;12:248–80.

52. Sala E, Rockall AG, Freeman SJ, et al. The added role of MR imaging in treatment stratification of patients with gynecologic malignancies: what the radiologist needs to know. Radiology 2013;266(3): 717–40.

53. Ayhan A, Taskiran C, Celik C, et al. The long-term survival of women with surgical stage II endometrioid type endometrial cancer. Gynecol Oncol 2004;93(1):9–13.

54. Kakhki VR, Shahriari S, Treglia G, et al. Diagnostic performance of fluorine 18 fluorodeoxyglucose positron emission tomography imaging for detection of primary lesion and staging of endometrial cancer patients: systematic review and meta-analysis of the literature. Int J Gynecol Cancer 2013;23(9): 1536–43.

55. Lerman H, Metser U, Grisaru D, et al. Normal and abnormal 18F-FDG endometrial and ovarian uptake in pre- and postmenopausal patients: assessment by PET/CT. J Nucl Med 2004;45(2):266–71.

56. Liu Y. Benign ovarian and endometrial uptake on FDG PET-CT: patterns and pitfalls. Ann Nucl Med 2009;23(2):107–12.

57. Kinkel K, Kaji Y, Yu KK, et al. Radiologic staging in patients with endometrial cancer: a meta-analysis. Radiology 1999;212(3):711–8.

58. Bollineni VR, Ytre-Hauge S, Bollineni-Balabay O, et al. High diagnostic value of 18F-FDG PET/CT in endometrial cancer: systematic review and meta-analysis of the literature. J Nucl Med 2016;57:879–85.

59. Jung DC, Ju W, Choi HJ, et al. The validity of tumour diameter assessed by magnetic resonance imaging and gross specimen with regard to tumour volume in cervical cancer patients. Eur J Cancer 2008;44(11):1524–8.

60. Connor JP, Andrews JI, Anderson B, et al. Computed tomography in endometrial carcinoma. Obstet Gynecol 2000;95(5):692–6.

61. Manfredi R, Mirk P, Maresca G, et al. Local-regional staging of endometrial carcinoma: role of MR imaging in surgical planning. Radiology 2004;231(2):372–8.

62. Kitajima K, Murakami K, Yamasaki E, et al. Accuracy of integrated FDG-PET/contrast-enhanced CT in detecting pelvic and paraaortic lymph node metastasis in patients with uterine cancer. Eur Radiol 2009;19(6):1529–36.

63. Signorelli M, Guerra L, Buda A, et al. Role of the integrated FDG PET/CT in the surgical management of patients with high risk clinical early stage endometrial cancer: detection of pelvic nodal metastases. Gynecol Oncol 2009;115(2):231–5.

64. Kadkhodayan S, Shahriari S, Treglia G, et al. Accuracy of 18F-FDG PET imaging in the follow up of endometrial cancer patients: systematic review and meta-analysis of the literature. Gynecol Oncol 2013;128(2):397–404.

65. Barwick TD, Rockall AG, Barton DP, et al. Imaging of endometrial adenocarcinoma. Clin Radiol 2006;61(7):545–55.

66. Sala E, Wakely S, Senior E, et al. MRI of malignant neoplasms of the uterine corpus and cervix. AJR Am J Roentgenol 2007;188(6):1577–87.

67. Rockall AG, Meroni R, Sohaib SA, et al. Evaluation of endometrial carcinoma on magnetic resonance imaging. Int J Gynecol Cancer 2007;17(1):188–96.

68. Frei KA, Kinkel K, Bonel HM, et al. Prediction of deep myometrial invasion in patients with endometrial cancer: clinical utility of contrast-enhanced MR imaging-a meta-analysis and Bayesian analysis. Radiology 2000;216(2):444–9.

69. Ascher SM, Reinhold C. Imaging of cancer of the endometrium. Radiol Clin North Am 2002;40(3):563–76.

70. Kitajima K, Suenaga Y, Ueno Y, et al. Value of fusion of PET and MRI for staging of endometrial cancer: comparison with (18)F-FDG contrast-enhanced PET/CT and dynamic contrast-enhanced pelvic MRI. Eur J Radiol 2013;82(10):1672–6.

71. Hennessy BT, Coleman RL, Markman M. Ovarian cancer. Lancet 2009;374(9698):1371–82.

72. Cannistra SA. Cancer of the ovary. N Engl J Med 2004;351(24):2519–29.

73. Angioli R, Plotti F, Capriglione S, et al. The role of novel biomarker HE4 in endometrial cancer: a case control prospective study. Tumour Biol 2013;34(1):571–6.

74. Morgan RJ. Ovarian cancer guidelines: treatment progress and controversies. J Natl Compr Canc Netw 2011;9:4–5.

75. Morgan RJ Jr, Alvarez RD, Armstrong DK, et al. Ovarian cancer, version 3.2012. J Natl Compr Canc Netw 2012;10:1339–49.

76. Morgan RJ, Alvarez RD, Armstrong DK, et al. Ovarian cancer, version 2.2013. J Natl Compr Canc Netw 2013;11:1199–209.

77. Nam EJ, Yun MJ, Oh YT, et al. Diagnosis and staging of primary ovarian cancer: correlation between PET/CT, Doppler US, and CT or MRI. Gynecol Oncol 2010;116(3):389–94.

78. Agodi A, Barchitta M, Quattrocchi A, et al. DAPK1 promoter methylation and cervical cancer risk: a systematic review and a meta-analysis. PLoS One 2015;10(8):e0135078.

79. Tempany CM, Zou KH, Silverman SG, et al. Staging of advanced ovarian cancer: comparison of imaging modalities–report from the Radiological Diagnostic Oncology Group. Radiology 2000;215(3):761–7.

80. Grueneisen J, Schaarschmidt BM, Heubner M, et al. Implementation of FAST-PET/MRI for whole-body staging of female patients with recurrent pelvic malignancies: a comparison to PET/CT. Eur J Radiol 2015;84(11):2097–102.

81. Kitajima K, Suenaga Y, Ueno Y, et al. Value of fusion of PET and MRI in the detection of intra-pelvic recurrence of gynecological tumor: comparison with 18F-FDG contrast-enhanced PET/CT and pelvic MRI. Ann Nucl Med 2014;28(1):25–32.

Clinical PET/MR Imaging in Dementia and Neuro-Oncology

Otto M. Henriksen, MD, PhD,
Lisbeth Marner, MD, PhD, DMSc, Ian Law, MD, PhD, DMSc*

KEYWORDS

• PET/MR imaging • Dementia • Brain tumor • Glioma • Alzheimer disease

KEY POINTS

• PET/MR imaging using [18F]-fluorodeoxyglucose (FDG) is a practical clinical tool in the evaluation of dementia and allows for a fast, condensed, and well-accepted high-quality imaging protocol with interpretation effectively supported by statistical tools.

• In neuro-oncology, PET/MR imaging using [18F]-fluoro-ethyl-tyrosine (FET) is a practical clinical tool that can be adapted to different clinical demands depending on the clinical question.

• The clinical value of the multiparametric imaging capabilities of PET/MR imaging needs to be established.

INTRODUCTION

Commercially available integrated PET/MR imaging has recently been introduced in clinical nuclear medicine. Although it has been the cause of considerable excitement, the exact role and benefits of this technique have not been firmly defined. Given the key role that MR imaging has in the diagnostic evaluation of diseases of the brain, this application is an obvious clinical target to consider. The strength of MR imaging is the ability to perform detailed regional tissue characterization in high resolution and with superior soft tissue contrast. This is achieved through a time-consuming multisequence approach. Thus, as opposed to whole-body PET/MR imaging, in which MR imaging acquisition time is expended on screening body areas that may not be afflicted with disease using only a limited number of the most basic MR imaging sequences, acquisition time in PET/MR imaging of the brain is much more efficiently used for characterizing the organ

of interest. Ideally, the PET and MR imaging acquisitions are performed simultaneously to minimize total scanner time that may adversely affect image quality because of head movements. The patient groups that will have access to clinical PET/MR imaging are determined by local demands and procedures, prevalence of disease, the proven efficacy and availability of MR imaging sequences, PET radiotracers, work flow, and reimbursement. At our unit, dementia and brain tumors are the 2 primary indications for PET/MR imaging of the brain, constituting 75% and 25% of indications, respectively (**Fig. 1**).

There are a number of recent reviews presenting a broad perspective of possible PET/MR imaging applications for brain PET/MR imaging.[1–5] These are not repeated in this review. It is possible to perform very lengthy MR imaging acquisitions that may be considered experimental without established clinical value for the patient. Instead, we present the experiences and diagnostic

The authors have nothing to disclose.
Department of Clinical Physiology, Nuclear Medicine & PET, Rigshospitalet, 9, Blegdamsvej, Copenhagen 2100-DK, Denmark
* Corresponding author.
E-mail address: ilaw@dadlnet.dk

Clinical Brain PET/MRI Production: 2013–2015

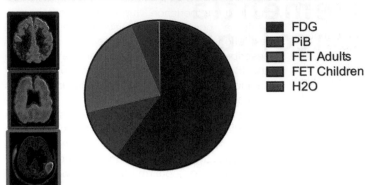

■ FDG
■ PiB
■ FET Adults
■ FET Children
■ H2O

Total = 937 (47% of all PET/MRI)

Fig. 1. Distribution of clinical PET/MR imaging brain studies. Pie plot showing the distribution of clinical PET/MR imaging brain studies over a 3-year period divided by PET radiotracer. Brain studies constitute approximately 50% of all scans performed, and is dominated by patients referred for neurodegeneration (3/4, FDG or PiB) and neuro oncology (1/4, FET).

strategies used from the realities of a single institution based on immediate clinical value.

PET/MR IMAGING IN DEMENTIA

The dementias are dominated by neurodegenerative disease and cerebrovascular disease (CVD). Most neurodegenerative diseases are histologically characterized by the progressive accumulation of protein structures of low solubility in brain tissue, and the progressive destruction of neural tissue. The most common neurodegenerative disease is Alzheimer disease (AD), which accounts for approximately 50% of all patients with dementia, whereas CVD is the cause of 30% of dementia cases, vascular cognitive disorder (VCD),[6] where half of these cases also have AD pathology (mixed dementia). Other causes are Lewy body dementia (DLB) and fronto-temporal lobar degeneration (FTLD), each with their own distinctive pathology.

Brain Imaging in Dementia

Accurate and early diagnosis is central to the management of patients suffering from neurodegenerative disease. Both PET and MR imaging are established clinical tools that to a large extent give independent and complementary clinically valuable information. The functions that a series of MR imaging sequences should be able to contain to support PET interpretation and to exclude or identify clinically relevant pathologic conditions are listed in **Box 1**. A standard MR imaging clinical dementia protocol will usually consist of variations of the 4 sequences in **Box 2**. Initially, a Dixon water-fat-separation (DWFS) sequence is usually performed and/or the ultrashort echo time (UTE) sequences that some use for attenuation correction (AC). Thus, a relatively lean less than 20-minute MR imaging

session composed of the essential sequences contributes most value to the routine clinical evaluation of the patient with general dementia. Two optional sequences to consider are diffusion-weighted imaging (DWI) and three-dimensional (3D) postcontrast T1-weighted magnetization-prepared rapid gradient echo (T1-MPRAGE) in the complicated patient (see **Box 2**). In our setting, the more unusual clinical presentation will lead to the relevant MR imaging sequences performed before PET. Thus, DWI or 3D postcontrast T1-MPRAGE is performed by request only or post hoc in a separate MR imaging session for this

---

Box 1
Most important uses of MR imaging in clinical PET/MR imaging of dementia

- Exclude structural lesions that may be treated neurosurgically: subdural hematoma, brain tumor (meningioma, metastasis, glioma), arteriovenous malformation, normal-pressure hydrocephalus.

- Exclude generalized or local edema; for example, secondary to infection/inflammation (encephalitis, Creutzfeldt-Jakob disease).

- Identify cerebrovascular pathology: vascular white matter lesions, territorial infarcts, lacunar infarcts, (micro) hemorrhages.

- Identify other structural lesions or abnormalities of importance: regional cortical and central atrophy,[a] hippocampal atrophy, trauma, developmental disorders (heterotopia).

- Facilitate integration of the above in the evaluation of the local and distant functional effects of structural change.

[a] This includes a widening of the perivascular Virchow-Robin spaces.

Box 2
An MR imaging clinical dementia protocol

Standard:

- Three-dimensional (3D) T1-weighted magnetization-prepared rapid acquisition gradient-echo (T1-MPRAGE) sequence (5 minutes) is particularly well suited for evaluation of structural pathology and regional atrophy, for example, of the hippocampal structures.

- T2-weighted fluid attenuation inversion recovery (FLAIR) sequence (2.5 minutes) and T2-weighted BLADE or turbo spin-echo (TSE) sequence (1.5 minutes) are sensitive for detection of edema, demyelination, and ischemic changes, and are important in identifying neoplasms and cerebrovascular disease.

- Susceptibility-weighted imaging (SWI) sequence or gradient-echo T2*-weighted sequence (6 minutes) are sensitive to blood products and are useful to identify cerebral hemorrhage. Microbleeds (<5 mm) may be found in hypertensive patients in the basal ganglia, thalami, or posterior fossa. If the microbleeds are lobar and corticomedullary in location, this indicates cerebral amyloid angiopathy.

Optional:

- Diffusion-weighted imaging (DWI) (4 minutes): younger patients, rapidly progressive dementia, suspicion of infection, including Creutzfeldt-Jakob disease, vasculitis, tumor, and recent infarct (<3 weeks).

- 3D postcontrast T1-MPRAGE: rapidly progressive dementia, suspicion of infection, tumor, and vasculitis.

---

purpose if indicated by our initial MR imaging evaluation.

PET Radiotracers in Dementia

The most relevant PET radiotracers are [18F]-fluorodeoxyglucose (FDG), and the amyloid tracers: [11C]-Pittsburgh compound B (PiB), [18F]florbetapir, [18F]florbetaben, and [18F] flutemetamol. In our setting, FDG is the primary clinical dementia radiotracer. FDG PET provides a measure of relative regional glucose metabolism, which is an indirect measure of synaptic function. FDG uptake is reduced with loss of neural activity; for example, in loss of viable neurons or in functional deactivation (diaschisis). FDG is widely available, driven by the demands in oncology, relatively cheap, and requires only a short 10-minute PET acquisition. FDG PET has a high diagnostic accuracy in distinguishing AD from healthy controls or other neurodegenerative conditions, such as FTD,[7] and in identifying patients with mild cognitive impairment (MCI) that will convert to AD.[8] Furthermore, FDG PET imaging is accepted as a neuronal injury imaging biomarker as recommended by the National Institute on Aging and the Alzheimer's Association work group,[9] and as an AD progression marker according to the International Working Group (IWG) for New Research Criteria for the Diagnosis of Alzheimer's Disease.[10]

The amyloid binding radiotracers are also integrated into the previously discussed two recommendations identifying a necessary etiologic prerequisite of AD. However, we find the amyloid radiotracers to be less useful in the clinical routine than FDG. Increased amyloid binding constitutes a risk factor that may appear decades before symptom onset.[11] However, a negative amyloid PET scan does not exclude neurodegeneration by other causes, costs are higher, and its availability lower. Thus, if we find AD typical parieto-temporal metabolic deficits that cannot be explained by structural lesions, we need not proceed further. Amyloid imaging is largely used as a supplementary investigation if FDG PET results are ambiguous (**Fig. 2**).

Clinical Work Flow and Clinical Use

Our standard 20 minute PET/MR imaging clinical protocol is composed of 4 standard MR imaging sequences (see **Box 2**) and a simultaneous 10-minute PET acquisition performed 40 minutes after injection of 200 MBq FDG (see **Fig. 2**) according to guidelines.[12,13] This short PET/MR imaging protocol is well suited for large-scale clinical throughput, and we find it a convenient and acceptable solution for patients and caregivers.

In a recent meta-analysis, it was shown that the diagnostic and prognostic accuracy of MR imaging and PET imaging AD biomarkers is at least as dependent on how the biomarker is measured as on the type of biomarker itself.[14] Thus, FDG PET performs best using statistical evaluation to a control group, particularly as statistical surface projections,[15] which is performed routinely using vendor-provided solutions (see **Fig. 2**). Similarly, T1-MPRAGE is routinely segmented using

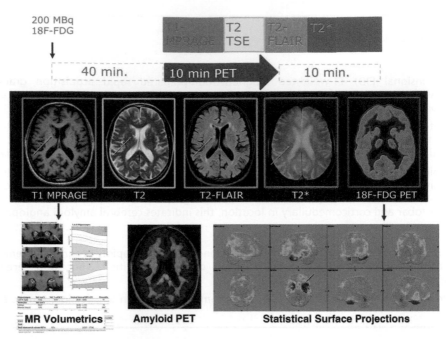

Fig. 2. PET/MR imaging brain protocol. Standard 20-minute FDG PET/MR brain imaging protocol consisting of 4 standard MR imaging sequences and FDG PET (top row) designed to identify the most common pathologies. This patient was initially diagnosed with semantic dementia, a variant of FTLD, but atypical AD was considered as a differential diagnosis. MR imaging identified a lacunar infarct in the internal capsule on the right side (*orange arrow*) and a single microbleed in the right thalamus (*green arrow*). Both abnormalities have minor or no effects on the regional metabolic activity seen in FDG PET. The hippocampal volumetric report (lower left) shows marked bilateral reduction in the total hippocampal volume (5.1 cm³) and a marked increase of the inferior lateral ventricular volume (4.9 cm³) with significant asymmetry, where the left hippocampal volume (*cyan arrow*) is only 70% of that on the right. FDG PET statistical surface projection maps (lower right) showed the same asymmetry in the anterior temporal lobes (*red arrow*), along with moderate to severe metabolic reduction extending posteriorly to involve the temporal and parietal lobes, including the posterior cingulate gyrus on the left. A supplementary amyloid PiB PET scan (*lower center*) was negative, indicating semantic dementia rather than atypical AD.

FreeSurfer,[16] generating an MR imaging volumetric measurement report with particular emphasis on the hippocampal volume (HPV) (see **Fig. 2**). This is superior to a visual score.[17] Although HPV has a smaller diagnostic accuracy than FDG PET,[14] this is a low-cost metric that may add to the overall diagnostic accuracy in identifying neuronal damage in neurodegeneration.[18] As approximately 30% of patients from a general dementia population can be expected to have VCD, it is very important in the PET image reading to be able to integrate functional and structural imaging correctly to label regional metabolic reductions as potentially caused by local or remote effects of structural damage or, if this is can be ruled out, to possible neurodegeneration (see **Fig. 2**).

Future Developments in Dementia

There are a number of advanced MR imaging techniques that may contribute to the diagnosis of the

individual patients.[4] Arterial spin labeling (ASL) can measure regional cerebral blood flow (rCBF) by magnetically tagging the arterial water proton spins using dedicated pulse sequences followed by kinetic modeling. The perspective would be to substitute FDG PET by ASL MR imaging, and good correlation has been found in a number of publications.[19,20] These are intriguing findings, and although a white paper has been published recommending one ASL version, pseudocontinuous ASL,[21] neither harmonized MR imaging sequences nor postprocessing strategies are available for all MR imaging platforms. As the half-life of the magnetic tag is very short, ASL is signal-to-noise limited and the rCBF distribution critically dependent on arrival time. Late bolus arrival will be found as a consequence of CVD or in the watershed areas, for example, in parietotemporal cortex, and may mimic an AD pattern in healthy subjects.[19] Thus, rigid clinical evaluation is essential and PET/MR imaging provides the ideal tool for this.

PET/MR IMAGING IN NEURO-ONCOLOGY

Imaging plays a pivotal role in the management of all brain tumors, including the initial diagnostic workup and planning of therapy, therapy monitoring, and detection of residual or recurrent disease. Tumors of the central nervous system comprise a heterogeneous group of neoplasms. In adults, glioblastoma multiforme (GBM) (World Health Organization [WHO] grade IV) is the most common primary malignant brain tumor,[22] and is associated with a median survival of 15 months despite optimal surgery and standard radiochemotherapy.[23]

Central nervous system tumors are the most common solid tumors in children,[24] with medulloblastoma and low-grade glioma being the most frequent pathologies.[22] As opposed to adult brain tumors, pediatric brain tumors are more often located in the posterior fossa and medulla, and show the highest incidences of death and late-life disability related to childhood cancers.[24–26]

The primary aim of imaging in neuro-oncology is to correctly separate tumor from normal brain tissue, treatment-induced changes, and other pathologies. MR imaging is considered the standard imaging modality, but various PET radiotracers and advanced MR imaging techniques are increasingly being used in all stages of the disease as a supplement to MR imaging. Hybrid PET/MR imaging systems thus offer the possibility of single-session multiparametric imaging by combining basic and advanced MR imaging techniques and any available PET radiotracer with the aim of improving overall diagnostic accuracy. In the following sections, currently used MR imaging and PET techniques applied in neuro-oncology are briefly reviewed with particular emphasis on imaging of gliomas.

MR Imaging for Brain Tumors

Standard MR imaging protocols for brain tumors generally include the same sequences as those used for neurodegenerative diseases (see **Box 2**): T2-weighted and fluid attenuation inversion recovery (FLAIR) sequences visualizing nonenhancing infiltrating tumor components, edema, and therapy-induced gliosis, and a 3D postcontrast T1-weighted sequence depicting tumor angiogenesis and contrast agent leakage. A precontrast T1-weighted sequence also may be useful to separate contrast enhancement from blood products. The standard protocol may be supplemented by susceptibility-weighted imaging (SWI) or T2*-weighted sequences showing blood products, and DWI to identify areas of restricted motion (ie, decreased apparent diffusion coefficient [ADC]) of water molecules due to acute infarction and to separate tumor from abscess. Reduced ADC may also be used to identify areas of increased cellularity in tumors.[27]

Dynamic T2*-weighted (dynamic susceptibility contrast [DSC]) or T1-weighted (dynamic contrast-enhanced [DCE]) imaging during bolus passage of a gadolinium-based contrast agent may be used to assess tumor blood volume (BV) as a marker of neoangiogenesis and malignancy, and may also provide information on tumor blood flow and leakage.[28]

Proton magnetic resonance spectroscopy (1H-MRS) allows semiquantitative assessment of selected metabolites in conspicuous lesions. The most widely studied metabolites include choline reflecting increased cellular membrane synthesis, N-acetylaspartate as a marker of neuronal loss, and creatine as an internal standard. Increased ratios of choline/N-acetylaspartate and of choline/creatine are generally believed to indicate malignancy.[29]

PET Radiotracers for Neuro-Oncology

Assessment of tumor glucose metabolism by FDG has been widely used for brain tumor imaging, but due to the high physiologic uptake in the surrounding normal brain tissue, more selective radiotracers are increasingly being used.

PET imaging using radiolabeled amino acids, such as [11C]-methionine (MET), [18F]-fluoro-ethyl-tyrosine (FET), and [18F]-fluoro-phenylalanine (FDOPA), targeting the L-amino acid transporter type 1 and 2 systems, which are upregulated in neoplastic brain tissue, provides high tumor-to-background imaging.[30] This group of radiotracers is also transported across the intact blood-brain barrier, and is suitable for imaging of low-grade gliomas. The performance of all amino acid radiotracers for delineation of the metabolically active tumor volume is generally very similar, although 18F-labeled compounds may be preferred to 11C-labeled compounds due to the short half-life of 11C (20 minutes). For FET PET imaging, biopsy-verified tumor-to-background thresholds for separating tumor tissue from surrounding normal tissue have been established,[31] aiding image analysis. Unlike FDOPA and MET PET imaging, dynamic FET PET imaging may further provide time-activity curves, which have been shown to provide diagnostic information for tumor grading[32] and for evaluation of brain metastases following radiotherapy.[33] It should be noted though that increased radiotracer uptake above the standard threshold may also be observed in non-neoplastic lesions[34] as well as in reactive changes and astrogliosis, following surgery and radiotherapy.[35]

Amino acid PET radiotracers also show uptake in lymphomas and meningiomas, but for these indications other PET radiotracers are preferred, such as FDG and somatostatin receptor II binding ligands (such as [68Ga]-DOTATOC), respectively.[36]

Clinical Workflow

To allow PET/MR imaging to replace diagnostic MR imaging, we have implemented and adapted the MR imaging protocols of neuroradiology. For research use, various study-specific MR imaging sequences may be added within the duration of the PET scan.

Fig. 3 shows an example of a clinical protocol for treated high-grade gliomas from our institution using FET as radiotracer providing a comprehensive diagnostic evaluation within a 20-minute static PET scan commenced 20 minutes after injection of 200 MBq of FET. For metastases, low-grade gliomas, and in all pediatric patients, a 40-minute dynamic scan is performed following injection of the radiotracer in order to obtain additional information about the tracer-kinetics in the lesion as described previously. This also provides opportunity for additional MR imaging sequences (**Fig. 4**, top panel).

Pediatric brain tumors have a high risk of spreading to the spinal cord, and primary tumors in the spinal cord are more common in children. Thus, often the routine brain examination as described previously is supplemented by a spinal cord MR imaging protocol (see **Fig. 4**, lower panel). If suspicious lesions are identified, a transverse T1-weighted sequence is added combined with a 10-minute static PET scan. The very late acquisition of spinal cord PET images (70–90 minutes after radiotracer injection) excludes the possibility for any semiquantitative analysis of data but a visual inspection is still possible at this time point using FET. If the primary tumor is located in the spinal cord, we use a dynamic PET scan at the site of the known tumor combined with spinal cord MR imaging.

The pediatric patient group is more vulnerable with regard to diagnosis, treatment, and patient care. A combined PET/MR imaging scan is thus even more relevant in this age group, as two separate scanning procedures are more stressful for the young children and their parents. Especially in children younger than 8 years in whom anesthesia or sedation usually is required, a single-session PET/MR scan greatly reduces the stress and risks associated with separate scans (**Fig. 5**).

For children not requiring anesthesia, availability of a quiet and comforting atmosphere where the child and parents feel safe is mandatory. Slight sedation with tranquilizers (or feeding in infants) may induce sleep and improve the quality of the investigation. We additionally use an advanced 3D surface surveillance system[37] that enables real-time monitoring with quantitative registration of head movements. This may allow repetition of key MR imaging sequences within the scanning session or post hoc PET scan motion correction.

Clinical Use

Using various protocols, we have successfully performed nearly 300 combined brain FET and

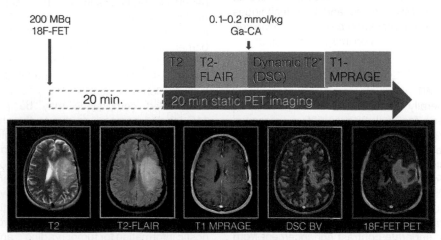

Fig. 3. Basic 20-minute static FET PET and MR imaging with DSC BV imaging. The injection of the contrast agent is combined with a DSC perfusion sequence that allows for the quantification of cerebral blood volume. After contrast injection, a T1-MPRAGE sequence concludes the session. The images show a patient with a nonenhancing WHO grade II oligodendroglioma receiving temozolomide. Note pronounced heterogeneity on both BV imaging and FET PET. (*From* Henriksen OM, Larsen VA, Muhic A, et al. Simultaneous evaluation of brain tumour metabolism, structure and blood volume using [(18)F]-fluoroethyltyrosine (FET) PET/MR imaging: feasibility, agreement and initial experience. Eur J Nucl Med Mol Imaging 2016;43(1):107, with permission.)

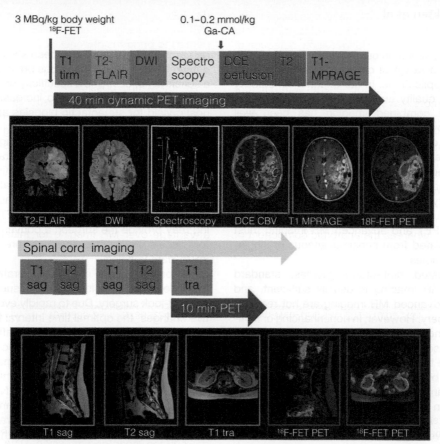

Fig. 4. Example of imaging protocol in pediatric neuro-oncology. A 40-minute dynamic PET simultaneous PET and MR imaging acquisition is started with the injection of 3 MBq/Kg body weight FET. If clinically relevant, the protocol can be supplemented with MR imaging of the spinal cord with transverse imaging and PET of suspicious lesions. Clinical images were obtained in 2 different patients: a 14-year-old girl with anaplastic glioma in her left hemisphere (*top row*) and a different 14-year-old girl with spinal metastasis (*red arrow*) from a glioblastoma (*lower row*).

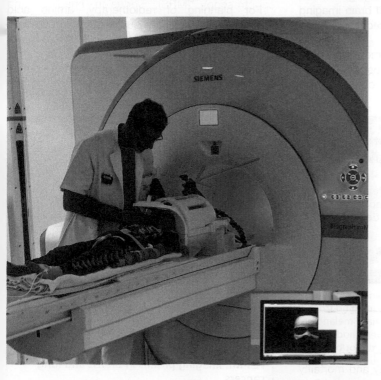

Fig. 5. Pediatric neuro-oncology PET/MR imaging imaging setup. An anesthetized child being prepared for a PET/MR imaging scanning procedure. Note the surface surveillance system (*red arrow*) attached to the head coil.

MR imaging scans on our hybrid PET/MR imaging system for a range of clinical indications and for research applications. In our experience, stability and image quality are similar to standalone systems, and combined imaging has been well accepted by both patients and caregivers.

PET and advanced MR imaging may be applied at all stages of disease. To date, most studies investigating the potential of simultaneous PET and MR imaging in neuro-oncology have focused on feasibility, whereas only very few have explored clinical value.[38,39] Therefore, most evidence on combined PET and advanced MR imaging must be extrapolated from nonsimultaneous or single-modality studies.

In untreated high-grade gliomas, standard anatomic MR imaging is usually sufficient, and PET and advanced MR imaging are not required before surgery. However, in nonenhancing or minimally enhancing lesions, and in patients with multifocal disease, advanced imaging techniques may be of value to assess tumor grade and to identify targets for biopsy.[40]

For dynamic FET PET, an accuracy of greater than 90% in adults for detection of high-grade gliomas was initially reported,[41] but more recent studies have suggested more modest values of approximately 80%,[42] and additional characterization may be valuable. Several studies have investigated the potential of combined amino acid PET and advanced MR imaging techniques including MRS, DWI, and BV imaging,[43,44] but the results are not consistent, and brain imaging cannot substitute for biopsy or resection with histologic tissue confirmation.

The use of amino acid PET and more advanced MR imaging techniques like spectroscopy in pediatric neuro-oncology is still subject of ongoing research.[45,46] MET PET has been shown to differentiate tumor from nontumorous brain lesions with a sensitivity of 83% and a specificity of 92%,[47] and MET PET has been shown to increase the diagnostic yield for stereotactic biopsies and surgical management (**Fig. 6**).[48]

Functional MR imaging (fMR imaging)[49] and diffusion-tensor imaging (DTI) tractography[50] may be applied to identify eloquent cortex (in particular motor and speech) and white matter tracts, respectively, to assess safe margins of tumor resection. In the clinical workflow, PET/MR imaging may provide the surgeon a convenient means for accelerated comprehensive pre-procedural up-to-date imaging.

The primary aim of early postoperative imaging is the detection of residual tumor tissue prompting second-look surgery. Due to rapidly evolving reactive changes, the optimal time interval for postoperative MR imaging is 24 to 48 hours after surgery. The protocol should include also precontrast T1-weighted, SWI or T2*-weighted imaging, and DWI to separate hemorrhage and infarcts from contrast-enhancing residual tumor. Neither PET nor advanced MR imaging techniques are routinely used in the early postoperative stage. Postoperative reactive changes with nontumor FET uptake are sometimes present already within 72 hours of surgery, but comparison to the preoperative MR imaging and preferably a preoperative FET PET can usually help distinguish the cause of FET uptake (**Fig. 7**).[51]

For planning of radiotherapy, amino acid PET may be used as a supplement to standard MR imaging to identify metabolically active tumor tissue outside standard margins around the MR imaging–based gross tumor volume to define the final target volume.[52] Often reactive uptake

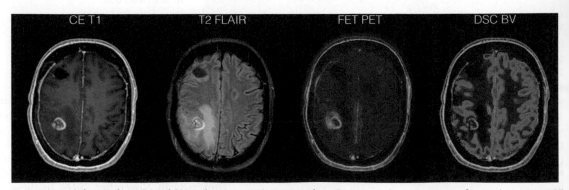

Fig. 6. Potential use of combined BV and amino acid PET imaging. Corresponding contrast-enhanced T1-MPRAGE (CE T1), T2 FLAIR, FET PET, and DSC BV imaging from 2 patients are presented. The patient had previously received stereotactic radiotherapy for a malignant melanoma metastasis in the right parietal region (and surgery in the right frontal region). FET PET showed moderately increased radiotracer uptake in the lateral part of the contrast-enhancing lesion (maximum tumor/background ratio = 2.5, mean tumor/background ratio = 1.8), but BV was not increased visually. Subsequent biopsy confirmed radionecrosis.

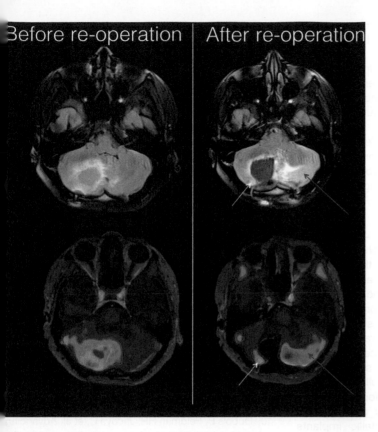

Fig. 7. Preoperative and postoperative PET/MR imaging. A 14-year-old girl presented with relapse of glioblastoma in right cerebellar hemisphere. Left: T2 FLAIR and FET PET before reoperation. Right: T2 FLAIR and FET PET 4 days after operation. Significant tumor remains (*white arrow*), and venous stasis after the surgical procedure is the likely cause of FET uptake in the left cerebellar hemisphere (*red arrow*). Careful reading using the preoperative FET PET/MR imaging as well as the increased signal intensity on the T2 FLAIR sequence is necessary to discriminate tumor from postoperative changes. MR imaging obtained 4 weeks later (not shown) supported the interpretation.

may be present, but to our knowledge no studies have investigated whether advanced MR imaging may be used to separate reactive FET uptake from tumor FET uptake. As computed tomography (CT) is mandatory for planning, PET/MR imaging offers no advantage over separate PET/CT and MR imaging in adults.

Response evaluation and detection of tumor recurrence are major challenges in neuro-oncology imaging. In patients with treatment-induced changes, in particular following radiotherapy or in patients exposed to antiangiogenic therapies, the diagnostic accuracy of standard MR imaging is compromised. Both amino acid PET and advanced MR imaging may be of value in this context.

BV imaging has been extensively studied for evaluation of tumor recurrence.[53] In treated gliomas, spatial congruence of amino acid PET and BV is generally poor, suggesting that the two modalities may provide complementary information.[54,55] Initial experience from our center has indicated that BV imaging may be of value in ambiguous FET PET lesions, such as moderately FET PET–positive BV-negative lesions that are less prone to progression on subsequent imaging favoring reactive changes.[54] A more recent study

including BV imaging, DWI, and MRS in addition to FET PET, showed that a combination FET PET and MRS (choline/creatine ratio) had the highest accuracy (97%) for separating radiation necrosis from tumor recurrence, whereas adding BV imaging and DWI did not improve the diagnostic accuracy.[38] However, the numbers of patients in both studies are very limited and further studies are needed, preferably with histologic confirmation.

Future Applications and Developments in Neuro-Oncology

Compared with PET imaging, MR imaging provides a large number of advanced imaging techniques. When designing the imaging protocol, one should carefully consider which parameters to obtain and analyze. Ideally, each parameter should provide complementary diagnostic information improving the diagnostic accuracy, but to date very few studies have investigated the diagnostic yield of multiparametric imaging in brain tumors. Also, the ability to actually use and incorporate the information may prove difficult, and for that purpose, image-processing software providing maps of combined parameters may be useful. Multiparametric imaging may be of particular value for investigating tumor heterogeneity, which could allow more targeted and personalized therapies.[56]

Finally, combining various MR imaging techniques with the novel PET radiotracers for imaging of tumor invasiveness, hypoxia, and proliferation could provide new insight into tumor biology, growth, and response to therapy.

In pediatric neuro-oncology, the development of silent MR imaging sequences, improved motion correction, and safe and more shallow anesthesia may ease the access to PET/MR imaging, resulting in improved diagnostics.

Limitations

In general, patients with claustrophobia, behavioral disturbances, or diseases of the spine and neck are ill suited for MR imaging, and should be referred to PET/CT scanning instead.

As the DWFS sequence for AC ignores bone, a systematic underestimation and strong spatial bias of radiotracer activity in the brain will occur. The vendor-provided UTE sequences do identify bone, but still suffer from errors in segmentation, resulting in discontinuities of the skull and misclassification of air/tissue interfaces, for example, in the sinuses.[57] In neuro-oncology patients with prior brain surgery, various metallic implants pose a particular challenge for AC of PET images when using MR imaging–based approaches. Thus, we routinely acquire separate low-dose CT scans of the head for AC in all of our clinical and research patients performed on the PET/MR imaging system.[58] These data have served as the basis for developing and testing CT independent attenuation strategies[59] that, however, must be rigidly tested clinically before clinical introduction.

The major limitation of clinical use of FET PET in pediatric neuro-oncology is the long acquisition time, especially when a spinal cord protocol is warranted. Head movements, lack of cooperation, discontinuation of the procedure due to discomfort, and the limited access to anesthesia are all major challenges when the patient is a younger child.

REFERENCES

1. Catana C, Drzezga A, Heiss WD, et al. PET/MRI for neurologic applications. J Nucl Med 2012;53(12): 1916–25.
2. Torigian DA, Zaidi H, Kwee TC, et al. PET/MR imaging: technical aspects and potential clinical applications. Radiology 2013;267(1):26–44.
3. Werner P, Barthel H, Drzezga A, et al. Current status and future role of brain PET/MRI in clinical and research settings. Eur J Nucl Med Mol Imaging 2015;42(3):512–26.
4. Barthel H, Schroeter ML, Hoffmann KT, et al. PET/MR in dementia and other neurodegenerative diseases. Semin Nucl Med 2015;45(3):224–33.
5. Yang ZL, Zhang LJ. PET/MRI of central nervous system: current status and future perspective. Eur Radiol 2016. [Epub ahead of print].
6. Sachdev P, Kalaria R, O'brien J, et al. Diagnostic criteria for vascular cognitive disorders: a VASCOG statement. Alzheimer Dis Assoc Disord 2014;28(3) 206–18.
7. Bohnen NI, Djang DS, Herholz K, et al. Effectiveness and safety of 18F-FDG PET in the evaluation of dementia: a review of the recent literature. J Nucl Med 2012;53(1):59–71.
8. Morbelli S, Brugnolo A, Bossert I, et al. Visual versus semi-quantitative analysis of 18F-FDG-PET in amnestic MCI: an European Alzheimer's Disease Consortium (EADC) project. J Alzheimers Dis 2015;44(3):815–26.
9. McKhann GM, Knopman DS, Chertkow H, et al. The diagnosis of dementia due to Alzheimer's disease: recommendations from the National Institute on Aging-Alzheimer's Association workgroups on diagnostic guidelines for Alzheimer's disease. Alzheimers Dement 2011;7(3):263–9.
10. Dubois B, Feldman HH, Jacova C, et al. Advancing research diagnostic criteria for Alzheimer's disease: the IWG-2 criteria. Lancet Neurol 2014; 13(6):614–29.
11. Jack CR Jr, Wiste HJ, Weigand SD, et al. Age-specific population frequencies of cerebral beta-amyloidosis and neurodegeneration among people with normal cognitive function aged 50-89 years: a cross-sectional study. Lancet Neurol 2014;13(10): 997–1005.
12. Waxman AD, Herholz K, Lewis D, et al. Society of Nuclear Medicine procedure guideline for FDG PET brain imaging version 1.0. 2009. Available at: http:// snmmi.files.cms-plus.com/docs/Society%20of%20 Nuclear%20Medicine%20Procedure%20Guideline %20for%20FDG%20PET%20Brain%20Imaging.pdf.
13. Varrone A, Asenbaum S, Vander BT, et al. EANM procedure guidelines for PET brain imaging using [18F]FDG, version 2. Eur J Nucl Med Mol Imaging 2009;36(12):2103–10.
14. Frisoni GB, Bocchetta M, Chetelat G, et al. Imaging markers for Alzheimer disease: which vs how. Neurology 2013;81(5):487–500.
15. Minoshima S, Frey KA, Koeppe RA, et al. A diagnostic approach in Alzheimer's disease using three-dimensional stereotactic surface projections of fluorine-18-FDG PET. J Nucl Med 1995;36(7):1238–48.
16. Fischl B. FreeSurfer. Neuroimage 2012;62(2):774–81.
17. Clerx L, Visser PJ, Verhey F, et al. New MRI markers for Alzheimer's disease: a meta-analysis of diffusion

tensor imaging and a comparison with medial temporal lobe measurements. J Alzheimers Dis 2012; 29(2):405–29.

18. Shaffer JL, Petrella JR, Sheldon FC, et al. Predicting cognitive decline in subjects at risk for Alzheimer disease by using combined cerebrospinal fluid, MR imaging, and PET biomarkers. Radiology 2013; 266(2):583–91.

19. Musiek ES, Chen Y, Korczykowski M, et al. Direct comparison of fluorodeoxyglucose positron emission tomography and arterial spin labeling magnetic resonance imaging in Alzheimer's disease. Alzheimers Dement 2012;8(1):51–9.

20. Verfaillie SC, Adriaanse SM, Binnewijzend MA, et al. Cerebral perfusion and glucose metabolism in Alzheimer's disease and frontotemporal dementia: two sides of the same coin? Eur Radiol 2015; 25(10):3050–9.

21. Alsop DC, Detre JA, Golay X, et al. Recommended implementation of arterial spin-labeled perfusion MRI for clinical applications: a consensus of the ISMRM perfusion study group and the European consortium for ASL in dementia. Magn Reson Med 2015;73(1):102–16.

22. Ostrom QT, Gittleman H, Fulop J, et al. CBTRUS Statistical Report: primary brain and central nervous system tumors diagnosed in the United States in 2008-2012. Neuro Oncol 2015;17(Suppl 4):iv1–62.

23. Stupp R, Mason WP, van den Bent MJ, et al. Radiotherapy plus concomitant and adjuvant temozolomide for glioblastoma. N Engl J Med 2005; 352(10):987–96.

24. Pollack IF, Jakacki RI. Childhood brain tumors: epidemiology, current management and future directions. Nat Rev Neurol 2011;7(9):495–506.

25. Pui CH, Gajjar AJ, Kane JR, et al. Challenging issues in pediatric oncology. Nat Rev Clin Oncol 2011;8(9): 540–9.

26. Koch SV, Kejs AM, Engholm G, et al. Educational attainment among survivors of childhood cancer: a population-based cohort study in Denmark. Br J Cancer 2004;91(5):923–8.

27. Sugahara T, Korogi Y, Kochi M, et al. Usefulness of diffusion-weighted MRI with echo-planar technique in the evaluation of cellularity in gliomas. J Magn Reson Imaging 1999;9(1):53–60.

28. Shiroishi MS, Castellazzi G, Boxerman JL, et al. Principles of T2 *-weighted dynamic susceptibility contrast MRI technique in brain tumor imaging. J Magn Reson Imaging 2015;41(2):296–313.

29. Martin NT, Sanchez-Gonzalez J, Martinez Barbero JP, et al. Clinical imaging of tumor metabolism with (1)H magnetic resonance spectroscopy. Magn Reson Imaging Clin N Am 2016;24(1):57–86.

30. Galldiks N, Langen KJ, Pope WB. From the clinician's point of view—what is the status quo of positron emission tomography in patients with brain tumors? Neuro Oncol 2015;17(11):1434–44.

31. Pauleit D, Floeth F, Hamacher K, et al. O-(2-[18F]fluoroethyl)-L-tyrosine PET combined with MRI improves the diagnostic assessment of cerebral gliomas. Brain 2005;128(Pt 3):678–87.

32. Popperl G, Kreth FW, Mehrkens JH, et al. FET PET for the evaluation of untreated gliomas: correlation of FET uptake and uptake kinetics with tumour grading. Eur J Nucl Med Mol Imaging 2007;34(12):1933–42.

33. Galldiks N, Stoffels G, Filss CP, et al. Role of O-(2-(18) F-fluoroethyl)-L-tyrosine PET for differentiation of local recurrent brain metastasis from radiation necrosis. J Nucl Med 2012;53(9):1367–74.

34. Hutterer M, Nowosielski M, Putzer D, et al. [18F]-fluoro-ethyl-L-tyrosine PET: a valuable diagnostic tool in neuro-oncology, but not all that glitters is glioma. Neuro Oncol 2013;15(3):341–51.

35. Popperl G, Gotz C, Rachinger W, et al. Value of O-(2-[18F]fluoroethyl)- L-tyrosine PET for the diagnosis of recurrent glioma. Eur J Nucl Med Mol Imaging 2004;31(11):1464–70.

36. Law I, Højgaard L. Brain tumors: other primary brain tumors, metastases and radiation injury. In: von Schulthess GK, editor. Clinical molecular anatomic imaging - PET/CT, PET/MR and SPECT/CT. Zürich: Wolters Kluwers Health; 2015. p. 169–79.

37. Olesen OV, Paulsen RR, Hojgaard L, et al. Motion tracking for medical imaging: a nonvisible structured light tracking approach. IEEE Trans Med Imaging 2012;31(1):79–87.

38. Jena A, Taneja S, Gambhir A, et al. Glioma recurrence versus radiation necrosis: single-session multiparametric approach using simultaneous O-(2–18F-Fluoroethyl)-L-Tyrosine PET/MRI. Clin Nucl Med 2016;41(5):e228–36.

39. Sacconi B, Raad RA, Lee J, et al. Concurrent functional and metabolic assessment of brain tumors using hybrid PET/MR imaging. J Neurooncol 2016; 127(2):287–93.

40. Jansen NL, Graute V, Armbruster L, et al. MRI-suspected low-grade glioma: is there a need to perform dynamic FET PET? Eur J Nucl Med Mol Imaging 2012;39(6):1021–9.

41. Popperl G, Kreth FW, Herms J, et al. Analysis of 18F-FET PET for grading of recurrent gliomas: is evaluation of uptake kinetics superior to standard methods? J Nucl Med 2006;47(3):393–403.

42. Albert NL, Winkelmann I, Suchorska B, et al. Early static F-FET-PET scans have a higher accuracy for glioma grading than the standard 20-40 min scans. Eur J Nucl Med Mol Imaging 2016;43(6):1105–14.

43. Floeth FW, Pauleit D, Wittsack HJ, et al. Multimodal metabolic imaging of cerebral gliomas: positron emission tomography with [18F]fluoroethyl-L-tyrosine and magnetic resonance spectroscopy. J Neurosurg 2005;102(2):318–27.

44. Bisdas S, Ritz R, Bender B, et al. Metabolic mapping of gliomas using hybrid MR-PET imaging: feasibility of the method and spatial distribution of metabolic changes. Invest Radiol 2013;48(5):295–301.

45. Law I, Borgwardt L, Højgaard L. Pediatric hybrid imaging of the brain. In: von Schulthess GK, editor. Clinical molecular anatomic imaging - PET/CT, PET/MR and SPECT/CT. Zürich: Wolters Kluwer Health; 2015. p. 218–29.

46. Dunkl V, Cleff C, Stoffels G, et al. The usefulness of dynamic O-(2-18F-fluoroethyl)-L-tyrosine PET in the clinical evaluation of brain tumors in children and adolescents. J Nucl Med 2015 Jan;56(1):88–92.

47. Galldiks N, Kracht LW, Berthold F, et al. [11C]-L-methionine positron emission tomography in the management of children and young adults with brain tumors. J Neurooncol 2010;96(2):231–9.

48. Pirotte BJ, Lubansu A, Massager N, et al. Results of positron emission tomography guidance and reassessment of the utility of and indications for stereotactic biopsy in children with infiltrative brainstem tumors. J Neurosurg 2007;107(5 Suppl):392–9.

49. Sunaert S. Presurgical planning for tumor resectioning. J Magn Reson Imaging 2006;23(6):887–905.

50. Potgieser AR, Wagemakers M, van Hulzen AL, et al. The role of diffusion tensor imaging in brain tumor surgery: a review of the literature. Clin Neurol Neurosurg 2014;124:51–8.

51. Marner L, Nysom K, Sehested A, et al. Feasibility of early postoperative 18F-FET PET/MRI after surgery for brain tumor in pediatric patients. ISPNO Conference Proceeding RA07; 2016.

52. Munck af Rosenschöld P, Costa J, Engelholm SA, et al. Impact of [18F]-fluoro-ethyl-tyrosine PET imaging on target definition for radiation therapy of high-grade glioma. Neuro Oncol 2015;17(5):757–63.

53. Bisdas S, Kirkpatrick M, Giglio P, et al. Cerebral blood volume measurements by perfusion-weighted MR imaging in gliomas: ready for prime time in predicting short-term outcome and recurrent disease? AJNR Am J Neuroradiol 2009;30(4):681–8.

54. Henriksen OM, Larsen VA, Muhic A, et al. Simultaneous evaluation of brain tumour metabolism, structure and blood volume using [(18)F]-fluoroethyltyrosine (FET) PET/MRI: feasibility, agreement and initial experience. Eur J Nucl Med Mol Imaging 2016;43(1):103–12.

55. Filss CP, Galldiks N, Stoffels G, et al. Comparison of 18F-FET PET and perfusion-weighted MR imaging: a PET/MR imaging hybrid study in patients with brain tumors. J Nucl Med 2014;55(4):540–5.

56. Reardon DA, Wen PY. Glioma in 2014: unravelling tumour heterogeneity-implications for therapy. Nat Rev Clin Oncol 2015;12(2):69–70.

57. Dickson JC, O'Meara C, Barnes A. A comparison of CT- and MR-based attenuation correction in neurological PET. Eur J Nucl Med Mol Imaging 2014; 41(6):1176–89.

58. Andersen FL, Ladefoged CN, Beyer T, et al. Combined PET/MR imaging in neurology: MR-based attenuation correction implies a strong spatial bias when ignoring bone. Neuroimage 2014;84:206–16.

59. Ladefoged CN, Benoit D, Law I, et al. Region specific optimization of continuous linear attenuation coefficients based on UTE (RESOLUTE): application to PET/MR brain imaging. Phys Med Biol 2015; 60(20):8047–65.

PET/MR Imaging in Musculoskeletal Disorders

Kim Francis Andersen, MD[a], Karl Erik Jensen, MD, DMSc[b],
Annika Loft, MD, PhD[a],*

KEYWORDS

- FDG • Infection • Inflammation • Metastasis • Musculoskeletal • PET/MR imaging • Sarcoma

KEY POINTS

- Imaging with hybrid PET/MR imaging will probably supersede current use of PET/computed tomography and/or MR imaging in many diagnostic assessments of both benign and malignant conditions of the musculoskeletal system.
- Acquiring anatomic, molecular, and functional data simultaneously seems advantageous in the diagnostic workup, treatment planning and monitoring, and follow-up of patients with musculoskeletal disorders.
- Future studies should identify new clinical indications and be designed to answer specific clinical questions with integration of sophisticated MR imaging sequences and various PET radiotracers.

INTRODUCTION

The possibility of combining excellent soft tissue contrast imaging from magnetic resonance imaging (MR imaging) and various functional imaging parameters from MR imaging and PET in the form of PET/MR imaging is promising, which could have an impact on clinical oncological and nononcological imaging in general. With the various possibilities in MR imaging due to a variety of acquisition sequences, hereby gaining other types of information beyond superior soft tissue contrast, it would be expected to also increase the diagnostic information in different cancers and other disease conditions. With no ionizing radiation burden from MR imaging, it is a desirable alternative to the computed tomography (CT) component in hybrid PET imaging, which is of great importance especially for the pediatric

population. Also the "one-stop-shop" approach could result in a lower number of cumulative studies and thereby improve workflow.

This article focuses on bone and soft tissue lesions, ranging from infectious and inflammatory diseases to primary bone/soft tissue tumors to metastatic disease of the musculoskeletal system.

PET/MR IMAGING IN MUSCULOSKELETAL MALIGNANCIES
Primary Malignant Bone and Soft Tissue Tumors

Bone sarcomas (BS) and soft tissue sarcomas (STS) comprise a rare group of tumors, which exhibit mesenchymal differentiation. Sarcomas only comprise approximately 1% of all cancers.[1] However, with reported 5-year mortality rates of up to 50%[2] and extensive diversity in terms of

The authors have nothing to disclose.
[a] Department of Clinical Physiology, Nuclear Medicine & PET, Rigshospitalet, Copenhagen University Hospital, Blegdamsvej 9, PET-3982, Copenhagen DK-2100, Denmark; [b] Department of Diagnostic Radiology, Rigshospitalet, Copenhagen University Hospital, Blegdamsvej 9, Section 3024, Copenhagen DK-2100, Denmark
* Corresponding author.
E-mail address: Annika.Loft.Jakobsen@regionh.dk

PET Clin 11 (2016) 453–463
http://dx.doi.org/10.1016/j.cpet.2016.05.007

tumor histology, metastatic potential, and outcome,[1,3,4] diagnosis and treatment of these patients are challenging. Consequently, the diagnostic workup requires a multimodal approach, and treatment protocols for patients with sarcoma include surgery, neoadjuvant and adjuvant chemotherapy, radiotherapy, and more recently strategies with targeted therapy.[5–8]

In sarcomas, both MR imaging and [18F]-2-fluoro-2-deoxy-D-glucose (FDG) PET/CT are routinely used, and the application of these imaging modalities is supported by strong data. For characterization of BS and STS, gadolinium-enhanced MR imaging is the current reference standard. Due to the superior soft tissue contrast and the ability to identify tumor involvement of soft tissue and neurovascular structures, as well as the extent of marrow changes,[9] the role of MR imaging in the identification, treatment planning (especially presurgical planning), and follow-up in patients with sarcoma is unique.

Sarcomas are heterogeneous and often present as large tumors at the time of diagnosis. As prognosis is strongly correlated with the histopathological tumor grade, representative tissue sampling is of importance, which may be guided by MR imaging.[4] With prolonged survival of patients with sarcoma due to the improved efficiency of surgery in combination with neoadjuvant and adjuvant chemotherapy/radiotherapy, the multiparametric imaging capabilities of MR imaging also have an increasing role both in treatment response monitoring as well as in the differentiation between posttreatment sequelae and residual/recurrent tumor tissue.[10] Finally, MR imaging does not expose patients to ionizing radiation, which is especially of importance in the younger patient population.

Based on the theory that malignant tissues tend to have high metabolic activity and as such accumulate the glucose analogue FDG to a higher degree than most normal tissues, metabolic imaging in terms of FDG PET has gained a significant role in the evaluation of many malignancies. In sarcomas, the application of metabolic imaging seems advantageous for large primary tumors and in cases with high tumor grade.[11] FDG PET as a standalone technique has demonstrated high sensitivity for detection of distant metastases on initial staging as well as for tumor recurrence in both BS and STS compared with conventional imaging modalities.[12–14] However, as standalone PET technology demonstrates inferior spatial resolution and capability of anatomic localization, a hybrid imaging modality with high-contrast and soft tissue resolution capability, such as CT and MR imaging, seems mandatory. Consequently, hybrid FDG PET/CT combines the high sensitivity of FDG PET for detection of the primary malignancy, malignant lymph nodes, and bone marrow metastases with the superior sensitivity of CT for detection of pulmonary malignant manifestations.[15] A number of studies have demonstrated the superior diagnostic performance, including impact on treatment strategy, of hybrid FDG PET/CT compared with either CT or FDG PET as standalone in staging and follow-up of patients with BS and STS.[11,16,17]

FDG PET has the ability to differentiate high-grade sarcomas from benign and low-grade tumors, as the degree of FDG uptake, semiquantitatively estimated in terms of standardized uptake value (SUV), correlates with histopathological tumor grade in sarcomas.[12,18,19] Thus, metabolic imaging has been shown to be helpful in planning a biopsy.[20] Representative tissue sampling minimizes the risk of underestimating tumor grade, which may affect prognostication as well as planning of therapy and follow-up in patients with sarcoma (**Fig. 1**). Furthermore, quantitative estimation of the FDG avidity can offer relevant information regarding the nature of the tumor, as SUV correlates with a number of histopathologic characteristics, response to neoadjuvant therapy, and clinical outcome.[21–25] More sophisticated quantitative FDG PET imaging markers in terms of metabolic tumor volume and total lesion glycolysis, which also take tumor burden and tumor heterogeneity into account, may add further knowledge for prognostication and therapy response evaluation in sarcomas.[26–29]

Benefits of PET/MR Imaging in Adult Sarcoma

Some of the advantages of hybrid PET/MR imaging in musculoskeletal malignancies are summarized in **Box 1** and more thoroughly described in recent reviews.[30,31] As previously mentioned, MR imaging is superior to CT in imaging tumors of the musculoskeletal system due to the limited soft tissue contrast of the latter imaging modality. Additionally, sophisticated MR imaging techniques allow a multiparametric characterization of tumor not available with CT. Thus, facilitated by the argument of a reduced exposure to ionizing radiation, an improved co-registration of PET and MR imaging data, as well as a possible reduction in overall imaging time, it is expected that the application of PET/MR imaging will supersede the use of PET/CT in the clinical setting of this tumor entity.[30,32]

PET/MR imaging could play a pivotal role in treatment planning and follow-up of patients with sarcoma. Although conventional MR imaging is the most versatile modality in musculoskeletal

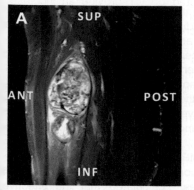
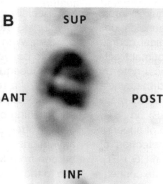
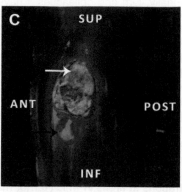

Fig. 1. Regional FDG PET/MR imaging assessment of the right thigh in a 73-year-old woman with a history of superficial spreading melanoma who presents with a rapidly growing right thigh mass. (*A*) Sagittal contrast-enhanced fat-suppressed T1-weighted spin-echo MR image demonstrates heterogeneous intramuscular mass with 2 major components located in right vastus intermedius muscle. (*B*) Sagittal FDG PET image and (*C*) fused sagittal FDG PET/MR image show inhomogeneous increased FDG uptake in superior component of mass (*white arrow*), and minimal FDG uptake in inferior component of mass (*black arrow*). The fused PET/MR imaging was used to guide biopsy from the most metabolically active part of the superior component. Histopathology demonstrated undifferentiated pleomorphic sarcoma, grade III (according to the French Federation of Cancer Centers Sarcoma Group (FNCLCC) grading system for adult STS). This patient was subsequently treated with tumor excision with marginal resection margins along with adjuvant radiation therapy. This case emphasizes the importance of representative tissue sampling, which minimizes the risk of underestimating tumor grade. This may affect prognostication as well as planning of therapy and follow-up in patients with musculoskeletal sarcoma. ANT, anterior; INF, inferior; POST, posterior; SUP, superior.

imaging, there are limitations concerning the exact definition of tumor infiltration into sites of peritumoral edema and adjacent structures. An overestimation of tumor volume and extension may result in major surgical intervention or amputation. Hence, a more specific imaging method in terms

---

Box 1
Advantages of hybrid PET/MR imaging

- Reduced exposure to ionizing radiation compared with PET/CT.
- High soft tissue contrast.
- Simultaneous multimodality imaging review.
- Advanced MR imaging sequences suited for multiparametric lesion characterization.
- Cross-validation of PET and MR imaging data may give additional valuable information.
- May reduce overall imaging time ("one-stop-shop").
- Provides more accurate co-registration.
- Robust MR imaging–based motion correction of PET data.

Data from Bashir U, Mallia A, Stirling J, et al. PET/MRI in oncological imaging: state of the art. Diagnostics (Basel) 2015;5(3):333–7; and Fraum TJ, Fowler KJ, McConathy J. PET/MRI: emerging clinical applications in oncology. Acad Radiol 2016;23(2):220–36.

---

of hybrid PET/MR imaging may reduce the morbidity following sarcoma surgery, an issue addressed by Loft and colleagues[33] in a case report. Additionally, in sarcomas in which radiation therapy is included in the treatment strategy, an improved tumor delineation by hybrid PET/MR imaging may be of importance due to the increasing tendency of image-guided intensity modulated radiotherapy with tight margins (ie, shrinkage of clinical target volumes and inverse-planned radiation).

In sarcomas, oncologic therapy monitoring and follow-up after treatment remain challenging. With an increasing number of patients undergoing targeted therapies and chemotherapeutic protocols with agents that exert unique modes of action (including cytostatic effects), there are still uncertainties regarding the best way to assess tumor response. Responding patients may demonstrate reduced tumor glucose metabolism on FDG PET as well as reduced tumor density, contrast enhancement, and changes in diffusion on MR imaging at an earlier stage than actual tumor size reduction.[21,34–36] Literature on the subject is sparse. However, there are small pilot studies and case reports demonstrating the feasibility of hybrid FDG PET/MR imaging for response assessment in sarcomas, in which the combined data were used by the clinicians in decision making in the neoadjuvant setting and to decide when to reinitiate chemotherapy. Also, the acquired information was used to resolve discrepancies between histologic grading and the clinical course of the disease, thus supporting the optimal treatment strategy.[37,38] Recently, a technical note by Zhang and colleagues[39] demonstrated the synergistic role of simultaneous PET/MR imaging–magnetic resonance spectroscopy (MRS) in STS metabolism imaging. The combination of superior soft tissue contrast (MR imaging), detection of enhanced tumor glucose metabolism (FDG PET), and specific information about metabolite concentrations at areas in which tumor may be difficult to differentiate from necrotic/inflammatory/fibrotic tissue (MRS), may yield an improved accuracy in treatment response assessment. An extension of this imaging concept has been introduced by Gutte and colleagues,[40] which demonstrated simultaneous FDG PET and MRS of hyperpolarized [13C]-pyruvate (hyperPET) in canine STS using a clinical hybrid PET/MR imaging system, offering a unique way of phenotyping tumor metabolism. As this approach could also be applicable for both image-guided surgical procedures and radiation therapy, guiding treatment with a boost radiation dose to residual areas of tumor, future investigations are expected.

Benefits of PET/MR Imaging in Pediatric Sarcoma

The major advantages of PET/MR imaging over PET/CT in pediatric sarcoma can be divided into the following[41]:

- Imaging-related benefits.
- Decreased exposure to ionizing radiation.
- Workflow optimization.

As in adult sarcoma, PET/MR imaging of sarcomas in a younger population combines the molecular information from the PET component with the superior soft tissue contrast, high-resolution, and multiparametric imaging capabilities of MR imaging in a single examination.[42] Potentially, a correlation of more advanced MR imaging sequences, such as diffusion-weighted imaging (DWI) and MRS with molecular-level metabolic PET data may give supplemental information for assessment of the tumors, influencing both planning and monitoring of treatment in pediatric sarcomas. Also, patient positioning during imaging may be a challenge in children. An improved imaging alignment has been achieved with hybrid PET/MR imaging compared with previous protocols fusing MR images with PET/CT data, as the risk of variance in patient positioning is higher in the latter scenario.

Especially in the pediatric population, the risk of developing radiation-related cancer is a major concern. With an established dose-response relationship between radiation dose during childhood and subsequent incidence of certain malignancies,[43] a reduction of ionizing radiation exposure may be the most important benefit of PET/MR imaging over PET/CT. Pediatric patients with cancer often undergo a number of diagnostic examinations,[44,45] and with no ionizing radiation burden from MR imaging, it is a desirable alternative to the CT component in hybrid imaging. Hirsch and colleagues[46] calculated that the effective dose of PET/MR imaging was only about 20% that of the equivalent PET/CT. Also, they postulated that the PET/MR imaging "one-stop-shop" approach used in their study resulted in a lower number of cumulative studies in their study population, consequently improving the workflow for pediatric patients in terms of decreased:

a. Ionizing radiation exposure.
b. Cumulative sedation time.
c. Associated stress level.
d. Delay in initiating therapy.

Combined PET/MR Protocols for Imaging of Sarcoma

The protocol selection for combined PET/MR imaging in sarcoma is a difficult challenge. First, one has to differentiate between whole-body imaging and separate anatomic compartment imaging, in which PET/MR imaging will be done only in a specific and limited anatomic area. The reduction in region of interest makes the composition of the combined PET/MR imaging protocol more feasible. Somehow, MR imaging data have to be acquired such that they can readily provide anatomic high-contrast images as well as attenuation maps. Because sarcomas only require regional imaging, PET/MR imaging could provide advantages over PET/CT. In these tumors, surrounding soft tissue infiltration is important for local staging as well as surgical and radiotherapy planning. Because of its higher soft tissue contrast, MR imaging has become the most significant morphologic modality for sarcoma imaging. Furthermore, treatment and workup of sarcomas have been highly centralized and standard MR imaging protocols have been established.

In Scandinavia, all patients referred for MR imaging of a possible bone or soft tissue tumor are examined with the protocol recommended by the Scandinavian Sarcoma Group (SSG).[47] This imaging protocol is simple, robust, and relative short in time consumption using only 5 MR imaging pulse sequences (**Box 2**). Time-saving PET/MR imaging

---

Box 2
The Scandinavian Sarcoma Group guidelines for basic MR imaging of suspected bone and soft tissue tumors

It is recommended that imaging of suspected tumors should be done on a high-field system ($\geq$1.0 T). The following sequences are recommended as a minimum. Additional sequences should be done according to local preferences.

1. Coronal short tau inversion recovery (STIR) sequence with large field of view for bone tumors, preferably covering 2 adjacent joints.

2. Axial T1-weighted spin-echo sequence (without fat suppression).

3. Axial T2-weighted fast/turbo spin-echo sequence (without fat suppression) with identical slice thickness and coverage as for the T1-weighted sequence.

Recommended sequences after intravenous injection of gadolinium-based contrast medium:

4. Axial T1-weighted spin-echo sequence, with identical imaging parameters as a precontrast sequence. If fat suppression is used, a precontrast fat-suppressed sequence is thus also needed.

5. If needed for further anatomic evaluation, a sagittal T1-weighted spin-echo sequence with fat suppression may be performed.

Adapted from The Scandinavian Sarcoma group guidelines for basic MRI of suspected bone and soft tissue tumours. 2012. Available at: http://www.ssg-org.net/wp-content/uploads/2011/05/Guidelines-for-basic-MRI-examination-of-suspected-bone-and-soft-tissue-tumors.pdf; with permission.

---

protocols are desirable, achieving the right compromise between the MR imaging sequences needed and a reasonable examination time, and then efficiently intercalating the acquired PET data and MR imaging sequences. The short SSG sarcoma MR imaging protocol has only to be combined with a Dixon-type pulse sequence (to provide the data for attenuation correction) and will allow for the simultaneous acquisition of PET data. A 2-point Dixon sequence produces water-weighted and fat-weighted images, and the image information of the acquired MR imaging data are used for tissue classification. Following this sequence, the image voxels can be segmented to tissue types, such as air, water, and fat, based on their MR imaging signal intensities.

One of the limitations of segmentation-based attenuation correction is that cortical bone is not accounted for by the standard Dixon method. As cortical bone attenuates PET photons more than soft tissue, an adequate signal is not provided to be represented in the attenuation correction maps derived from current MR imaging–based segmentation methods. Consequently, in tissues within or immediately adjacent to cortical bone, Aznar and colleagues[48] demonstrated lower quantitative estimations of FDG uptake in terms of SUV when assessed by PET/MR imaging compared with PET/CT. In general, even though specific data for sarcomas are lacking, the clinical impact of this underestimation of SUV (maximum reductions on the order of 10%–20%) on routine clinical imaging seems to be relatively minor.[31] There are

challenges to be solved with current extensive research into the subject.[49,50] Nevertheless, due to the short time consumption, this combined PET/MR imaging protocol even allows inclusion of a DWI sequence to investigate if it might be sufficient for follow-up on peritumoral edema in this patient population, especially when evaluating the apparent diffusion coefficient (ADC) values (**Fig. 2**). However, at this point, there is no established routine clinical staging and therapy follow-up protocol using PET/MR imaging in this setting.

Metastatic Disease of the Musculoskeletal System

Metastases are the most common malignant tumor involving osseous structures. After liver and lung, the skeleton is the third most involved site for metastases from carcinomas, the most common being prostate cancer in men and breast cancer in women, followed by lung cancer for both sexes.[51] Clinical complications of osseous metastases are pain, fractures, limited mobility, risk of spinal cord or nerve root compression, hypercalcemia, and bone marrow suppression, all of which need be considered in the treatment plan. Besides its impact on morbidity and quality of life, the presence of osseous metastases is also a prognostic factor.

Bone scintigraphy has been the method of choice for many years for detecting osseous metastases, especially for asymptomatic patients with moderate to high risk of developing metastases that give rise to increased local bone turnover.

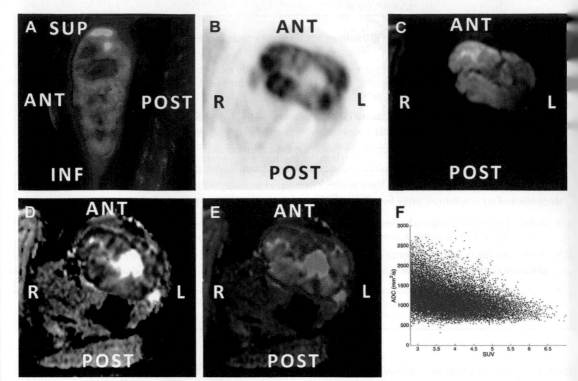

Fig. 2. Regional FDG PET/MR imaging assessment of the left thigh in a 70-year-old man with intramuscular un-differentiated pleomorphic sarcoma, grade III (FNCLCC). (*A*) Fused sagittal FDG PET image with sagittal contrast-enhanced fat-suppressed T1-weighted spin-echo MR image shows heterogeneous mass in vastus lateralis muscle with heterogeneous FDG uptake. (*B*) Transaxial FDG PET image again shows heterogeneous FDG uptake, predominantly in periphery of mass. (*C*) Transaxial DWI (b = 200) shows persistent areas of increased signal intensity, implying presence of viable tumor. (*D*) Transaxial ADC map image shows areas of low signal intensity, predominantly in periphery of mass, indicating presence of viable malignant tumor cells. (*E*) Fused transaxial FDG image with transaxial ADC map image shows similar findings as in (*C*) and (*D*). (*F*) Scatterplot demonstrates inverse correlation of ADC values with SUV. PET images were resampled to DWI resolution. An isocontour volume of interest (VOI) including all voxels above 40% of SUV_{max} was created for voxel-by-voxel analysis. Distinct distributions in the scatterplots of ADC versus SUV have the potential to be modeled so as to segment the tumor into distinct biologically relevant compartments, such as viable tumor tissue, inflammation, fibrosis, and necrosis. This case demonstrates the synergistic potential of hybrid PET/MR imaging in terms of acquiring anatomic, molecular, and functional data simultaneously. ANT, anterior; INF, inferior; L, left; POST, posterior; R, right; SUP, superior.

Due to its low spatial resolution and the fact that some tumors such as lymphoma and renal cell carcinoma cause isolated bone marrow infiltration or osteolytic metastases without any or only very little activation of normal bone turnover, the sensitivity and specificity for this method are 78% to 86% and 48% to 81%, respectively.[52,53] Bone scintigraphy is widely used also due to availability and the possibility to image the whole skeleton in one examination. PET/CT has as higher spatial resolution compared with bone scintigraphy. PET/CT using the radiotracers FDG or [18F]-labeled sodium fluoride ([18F]-NaF) has been shown to have higher sensitivities (90%–98% vs 56%–97%) and specificities (100% vs 97%) in detecting osseous metastases compared with bone scintigraphy.[52,53]

MR imaging is a highly sensitive imaging method with high spatial and soft tissue resolution that provides the capability to reveal intramedullary metastases before cortical destruction occurs. Whole-body MR imaging techniques for detection of bone marrow metastases are becoming more widely available with sensitivity and specificity of 91% to 95% and 90% to 95%, respectively.[54,55]

The combination of metabolic information and high soft tissue contrast in FDG PET/MR imaging has been proposed for investigation of osseous lesions, and a few prospective studies have already been performed. Beiderwellen and colleagues[56] compared FDG PET/MR imaging with FDG PET/CT in 67 oncological patients with various primary tumors to assess osseous metastases by using PET/CT 60 minutes after FDG administration and a subsequent PET/MR imaging 152 minutes after FDG administration. They compared the conspicuity of lesions as well as the diagnostic confidence levels. PET/CT and PET/MR imaging were both found to be high-quality diagnostic tools for assessment of osseous metastases in a whole-body staging approach, with PET/MR imaging providing superior lesion conspicuity for osseous metastases and enabling the delineation of more malignant lesions than PET/CT, especially for small metastases. A possible weakness of the study is the time delay between PET/CT and PET/MR imaging in favor of a longer uptake time for FDG in the PET/MR imaging scans, thereby increasing the detection rate due to dual time point effects more than the imaging method itself. In a publication from 2015, Samarin and colleagues[57]

also looked at lesion conspicuity and reader confidence in 24 patients with 86 lesions. They found a similar overall detection rate for FDG PET/CT and PET/MR imaging, although the latter imaging modality had a higher reader confidence in interpretation of osseous lesions.

These results are in agreement with the conclusions of several retrospective studies and meta-analyses, the vast majority performed with FDG,[58] but results from studies using Gallium-68 [68Ga]-prostate specific membrane antigen (PSMA) for prostate cancer metastases have also been reported.[59] The high sensitivities found with [18F]-NaF PET combined with high resolution in MR imaging and its capability of detecting small bone marrow lesions (**Fig. 3**) is currently being investigated (Löfgren, personal report, 2016).

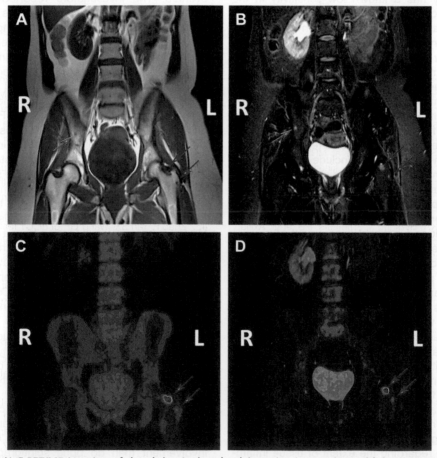

Fig. 3. [18F]-NaF PET/MR imaging of the abdominal and pelvic region in a patient with known prostate cancer referred for staging assessment. (*A*) Coronal T1-weighted spin-echo MR image and (*B*) coronal STIR MR image show 3 osseous metastases (*arrows*) involving the proximal left femur and right iliac bone. (*C*) Coronal [18F]-NaF PET maximum intensity projection image and (*D*) fused coronal [18F]-NaF PET/STIR MR image show concordance between both imaging modalities for the presence of the 2 proximal left femoral bone lesions (*red arrows*), but discordance for the presence of the right iliac bone lesion, which is detected on MR imaging but not on [18F]-NaF PET (*yellow arrow*) given its small size. This case illustrates the added value of combined PET and MR imaging modalities. L, left; R, right.

In summary, PET/MR imaging with FDG or ^{68}Ga-PSMA seems to have similar or even higher detection rates of metastatic osseous lesions with higher reader confidence than PET/CT, and hence could be more widely used in the clinical setting in the future. The main focus of studies involving PET/CT and a subsequent PET/MR imaging has been the detection of lesions in the skeleton, whilst studies focusing on multiparametric imaging for improving diagnosis are yet to be performed.

PET/MR IMAGING IN INFLAMMATORY AND INFECTIOUS MUSCULOSKELETAL DISORDERS

The clinical imaging assessment of inflammatory disease has been limited to conventional radiography, assisting in the diagnosis and monitoring of disease progress. However, conventional radiography has a known low sensitivity in the detection of disease in the initial stages of tissue inflammation. The modern early anti-inflammatory treatment strategy uses drugs that significantly decrease the progression of the systemic inflammatory process. Therefore, an early diagnosis and an adequate follow-up of disease have become major challenges for radiology, and better results could be achieved if technologies combining functional as well as anatomic principles are used. Nuclear medicine techniques using Technetium-99m (99mTc) include 2-dimensional planar scintigraphy and 3-dimensional single-photon emission computed tomography, the latter of which permits reconstruction of images in sagittal, coronal, and axial planes.[60–62] Scintigraphy provides functional assessment of physiologic processes and therefore has significant potential for adequate follow-up of disease, although it provides poor anatomic visualization. A PET examination with the glucose analogue FDG allows for direct evaluation of tissue metabolism. It is well known that FDG accumulation occurs in inflammatory and infectious tissues. FDG uptake is based on an increased radiotracer accumulation within leukocytes, which use glucose after becoming activated. Contrast-enhanced MR imaging is the current reference standard in the diagnosis and follow-up of inflammatory and infectious musculoskeletal disease conditions. MR imaging can provide detailed high-resolution information regarding the extent of tissue inflammation, but during treatment, some diagnostic difficulties have been reported. However, MR imaging and FDG PET are strongly correlated with clinical findings in the wrists in patients with rheumatoid arthritis, and permit actual quantification of synovial joint inflammation as well as detection of disease activity.[61,62]

Few reports have been published reporting data from PET/MR imaging examinations in inflammatory disease. Regarding arthritis, Tatsumi and colleagues[63] reported a preclinical technical study demonstrating the feasibility for imaging targets in the rat body by using FDG, [11C]-methionine, and [18F]-NaF in an integrated PET/MR imaging scanner for small animals. [18F]-NaF uptake was observed in all joints and bones except for the ribs. Localization of sites of [18F]-NaF uptake was provided by the simultaneous MR imaging. A study by Fuchs and colleagues[64] was more focused on measuring cell proliferation noninvasively in vivo during different stages of experimental arthritis with [18F]-fluorothymidine (FLT) PET, but not with an integrated PET/MR imaging system. The animals were scanned on separate systems and the images were subsequently overlaid. The investigators reported increased radiotracer uptake in arthritic ankles compared with healthy ankles, where MR imaging was used for anatomic localization. An interesting case report was published by Chaudhari and colleagues[60] who performed PET/CT together with co-registered MR imaging before and after tumor necrosis factor (TNF)-alpha inhibitor therapy. Their initial results seemed to indicate that FDG uptake decreased in the sites of joint erosions.

Musculoskeletal infection may involve the appendicular and/or axial skeleton (osteomyelitis), the joint space (septic arthritis), or the soft tissues (cellulitis, myositis, fasciitis). Osteomyelitis is a broad group of infectious conditions that involve the bone and/or bone marrow. It can arise by hematogenous spread, via extension from a contiguous infection, or by direct inoculation during surgery or trauma. The diagnosis is not always clinically obvious, and imaging tests are frequently used to confirm and localize infected sites. Conventional bone scintigraphy is sensitive but not specific when underlying osseous pathology is present. Leukocyte scintigraphy is another nuclear medicine test used to diagnose osteomyelitis. This in vitro leukocyte labeling process is difficult and hampered by reduced diagnostic quality, and complementary bone marrow imaging is usually required to maximize diagnostic accuracy. MR imaging provides a more accurate and detailed visualization regarding the extent of disease involvement than do bone scintigraphy or CT. MR imaging with conventional T1-weighted, T2-weighted, and short tau inversion recovery (STIR) images normally permit differentiation of septic arthritis or soft tissue infection from osteomyelitis. Furthermore, contrast-enhanced MR imaging is capable of locating foci of active infection in areas of chronic osteomyelitis. Spondylodiscitis is presently the main manifestation of osteomyelitis. The initial diagnosis is often delayed due to nonspecific symptoms and a high prevalence of back pain. The diagnosis is based on clinical symptoms and signs, blood samples, and diagnostic imaging. MR imaging possesses good diagnostic sensitivity and specificity for the initial recognition of spondylodiscitis, but the evaluation of treatment response is currently poor. FDG PET/MR imaging may provide new information about tissue metabolism and thereby provide a possible method for direct noninvasive evaluation of antibiotic or surgical treatment. Similar diagnostic difficulties are present in diabetic patients with foot problems. Currently, a combination of scintigraphy, CT, and MR imaging is used to differentiate inflammation and/or neuropathic bone destruction from infection. FDG PET/MR imaging can provide anatomic detail with simultaneous metabolic data, and could be the method of choice in the future.

Musculoskeletal soft tissue infection usually manifests as hematogenous cellulitis/myositis or wound infection. Necrotizing fasciitis is the most severe kind of cellulitis (of bacterial origin), with bacterial spread along the deep fascia and muscles. Early recognition of this condition may be delayed by the nonspecific nature of the initial clinical signs and symptoms. Today, MR imaging is the most useful imaging modality in the diagnosis and delineation of necrotizing fasciitis. Contrast enhancement of the infected tissue and necrotic fascia can be variable, with a heterogeneous pattern of enhancement. Involvement of multiple anatomic compartments increases the likelihood of necrotizing fasciitis. No clinical trials have so far been reported, but PET/MR imaging may provide differentiating features from non-necrotizing soft tissue infections and inflammatory conditions, which may be hard clinically to differentiate from necrotizing fasciitis.

SUMMARY, CHALLENGES, AND FUTURE DIRECTIONS

Despite its promising future potential, hybrid PET/MR imaging still is relatively untested in clinical settings, and it remains unclear regarding exactly how important PET/MR imaging will be as a clinical diagnostic tool for the optimized evaluation of malignant and benign musculoskeletal disorders. To date, published data are often preclinical or based on small and heterogeneous patient cohorts, emphasizing the need for larger and more specifically designed studies to examine the synergistic potential of hybrid PET/MR imaging in terms of acquiring anatomic, molecular, and functional data simultaneously. There is a justified belief

that current challenges in terms of high machinery costs, technical issues (artifacts and quantitative inaccuracies), workflow-related issues, and a lack of harmonization in imaging guidelines will be solved, with emerging evidence suggesting that PET/MR imaging will have a role in many aspects of musculoskeletal imaging. Imaging protocols should, to a higher degree, be designed to answer specific clinical questions, to identify new clinical indications, and to determine which MR imaging sequences to combine with PET to give the most complementary information, adding value beyond what current imaging systems provide. Cross-validation of MR imaging and PET data may give additional valuable information, not only restricted to metabolism, but also of other biological hallmarks of musculoskeletal cancer and infection/inflammation, such as hypoxia, perfusion, and invasion. Consequently, the application of more sophisticated MR imaging sequences and other PET radiotracers beyond FDG in the diagnostic workup and follow-up of these patients should be explored.

ACKNOWLEDGMENTS

We are grateful to physicist Adam Espe Hansen, PhD, and Johan Löfgren, MD, for valuable help with figures.

REFERENCES

1. Fletcher CDM, Bridge JA, Hogendoorn PCW, et al. World Health Organisation classification of tumours of soft tissue and bone. 4th edition. Lyon (France): IARC Press; 2013.
2. Siegel R, Naishadham D, Jemal A. Cancer statistics, 2012. CA Cancer J Clin 2012;62(1):10–29.
3. Coindre JM, Terrier P, Guillou L, et al. Predictive value of grade for metastasis development in the main histologic types of adult soft tissue sarcomas: a study of 1240 patients from the French Federation of Cancer Centers Sarcoma Group. Cancer 2001; 91(10):1914–26.
4. Skubitz KM, D'Adamo DR. Sarcoma. Mayo Clin Proc 2007;82(11):1409–32.
5. Ballo MT, Ang KK. Radiation therapy for malignant melanoma. Surg Clin North Am 2003;83(2):323–42.
6. Ferrone ML, Raut CP. Modern surgical therapy: limb salvage and the role of amputation for extremity soft-tissue sarcomas. Surg Oncol Clin N Am 2012;21(2): 201–13.
7. Parida L, Fernandez-Pineda I, Uffman J, et al. Clinical management of Ewing sarcoma of the bones of the hands and feet: a retrospective single-institution review. J Pediatr Surg 2012; 47(10):1806–10.

8. Thompson PA, Chintagumpala M. Targeted therapy in bone and soft tissue sarcoma in children and adolescents. Curr Oncol Rep 2012;14(2):197–205.

9. Ilaslan H, Schils J, Nageotte W, et al. Clinical presentation and imaging of bone and soft-tissue sarcomas. Cleve Clin J Med 2010;77(Suppl 1):S2–7.

10. Partovi S, Chalian M, Fergus N, et al. Magnetic resonance/positron emission tomography (MR/PET) oncologic applications: bone and soft tissue sarcoma. Semin Roentgenol 2014;49(4):345–52.

11. Roberge D, Vakilian S, Alabed YZ, et al. FDG PET/CT in initial staging of adult soft-tissue sarcoma. Sarcoma 2012;2012:960194.

12. Charest M, Hickeson M, Lisbona R, et al. FDG PET/CT imaging in primary osseous and soft tissue sarcomas: a retrospective review of 212 cases. Eur J Nucl Med Mol Imaging 2009;36(12):1944–51.

13. Franzius C, Daldrup-Link HE, Wagner-Bohn A, et al. FDG-PET for detection of recurrences from malignant primary bone tumors: comparison with conventional imaging. Ann Oncol 2002;13(1):157–60.

14. Tateishi U, Yamaguchi U, Seki K, et al. Bone and soft-tissue sarcoma: preoperative staging with fluorine 18 fluorodeoxyglucose PET/CT and conventional imaging. Radiology 2007;245(3):839–47.

15. Volker T, Denecke T, Steffen I, et al. Positron emission tomography for staging of pediatric sarcoma patients: results of a prospective multicenter trial. J Clin Oncol 2007;25(34):5435–41.

16. Al-Ibraheem A, Buck AK, Benz MR, et al. (18) F-fluorodeoxyglucose positron emission tomography/computed tomography for the detection of recurrent bone and soft tissue sarcoma. Cancer 2013;119(6):1227–34.

17. Gerth HU, Juergens KU, Dirksen U, et al. Significant benefit of multimodal imaging: PET/CT compared with PET alone in staging and follow-up of patients with Ewing tumors. J Nucl Med 2007;48(12):1932–9.

18. Bastiaannet E, Groen H, Jager PL, et al. The value of FDG-PET in the detection, grading and response to therapy of soft tissue and bone sarcomas; a systematic review and meta-analysis. Cancer Treat Rev 2004;30(1):83–101.

19. Ioannidis JP, Lau J. 18F-FDG PET for the diagnosis and grading of soft-tissue sarcoma: a meta-analysis. J Nucl Med 2003;44(5):717–24.

20. Hain SF, O'Doherty MJ, Bingham J, et al. Can FDG PET be used to successfully direct preoperative biopsy of soft tissue tumours? Nucl Med Commun 2003;24(11):1139–43.

21. Benz MR, Czernin J, Allen-Auerbach MS, et al. FDG-PET/CT imaging predicts histopathologic treatment responses after the initial cycle of neoadjuvant chemotherapy in high-grade soft-tissue sarcomas. Clin Cancer Res 2009;15(8):2856–63.

22. Eary JF, O'Sullivan F, Powitan Y, et al. Sarcoma tumor FDG uptake measured by PET and patient outcome: a retrospective analysis. Eur J Nucl Med Mol Imaging 2002;29(9):1149–54.

23. Evilevitch V, Weber WA, Tap WD, et al. Reduction of glucose metabolic activity is more accurate than change in size at predicting histopathologic response to neoadjuvant therapy in high-grade soft-tissue sarcomas. Clin Cancer Res 2008;14(3):715–20.

24. Israel-Mardirosian N, Adler LP. Positron emission tomography of soft tissue sarcomas. Curr Opin Oncol 2003;15(4):327–30.

25. Kong CB, Byun BH, Lim I, et al. ^{18}F-FDG PET SUVmax as an indicator of histopathologic response after neoadjuvant chemotherapy in extremity osteosarcoma. Eur J Nucl Med Mol Imaging 2013;40(5):728–36.

26. Andersen KF, Fuglo HM, Rasmussen SH, et al. Volume-based F-18 FDG PET/CT imaging markers provide supplemental prognostic information to histologic grading in patients with high-grade bone or soft tissue sarcoma. Medicine 2015;94(51):e2319.

27. Benz MR, Allen-Auerbach MS, Eilber FC, et al. Combined assessment of metabolic and volumetric changes for assessment of tumor response in patients with soft-tissue sarcomas. J Nucl Med 2008;49(10):1579–84.

28. Choi ES, Ha SG, Kim HS, et al. Total lesion glycolysis by 18F-FDG PET/CT is a reliable predictor of prognosis in soft-tissue sarcoma. Eur J Nucl Med Mol Imaging 2013;40(12):1836–42.

29. Costelloe CM, Macapinlac HA, Madewell JE, et al. 18F-FDG PET/CT as an indicator of progression-free and overall survival in osteosarcoma. J Nucl Med 2009;50(3):340–7.

30. Bashir U, Mallia A, Stirling J, et al. PET/MRI in oncological imaging: state of the art. Diagnostics (Basel) 2015;5(3):333–57.

31. Fraum TJ, Fowler KJ, McConathy J. PET/MRI: emerging clinical applications in oncology. Acad Radiol 2016;23(2):220–36.

32. Czernin J, Ta L, Herrmann K. Does PET/MR imaging improve cancer assessments? Literature evidence from more than 900 patients. J Nucl Med 2014;55(Suppl 2):59S–62S.

33. Loft A, Jensen KE, Lofgren J, et al. PET/MRI for preoperative planning in patients with soft tissue sarcoma: a technical report of two patients. Case Rep Med 2013;2013:791078.

34. Forni C, Minuzzo M, Virdis E, et al. Trabectedin (ET-743) promotes differentiation in myxoid liposarcoma tumors. Mol Cancer Ther 2009;8(2):449–57.

35. Grosso F, Jones RL, Demetri GD, et al. Efficacy of trabectedin (ecteinascidin-743) in advanced pretreated myxoid liposarcomas: a retrospective study. Lancet Oncol 2007;8(7):595–602.

36. Bhojwani N, Szpakowski P, Partovi S, et al. Diffusion-weighted imaging in musculoskeletal radiology-clinical

applications and future directions. Quant Imaging Med Surg 2015;5(5):740–53.

37. Schuler MK, Platzek I, Beuthien-Baumann B, et al. (18)F-FDG PET/MRI for therapy response assessment in sarcoma: comparison of PET and MR imaging results. Clin Imaging 2015;39(5):866–70.

38. Schuler MK, Richter S, Beuthien-Baumann B, et al. PET/MRI imaging in high-risk sarcoma: first findings and solving clinical problems. Case Rep Oncol Med 2013;2013:793927.

39. Zhang X, Chen YL, Lim R, et al. Synergistic role of simultaneous PET/MRI-MRS in soft tissue sarcoma metabolism imaging. Magn Reson Imaging 2016; 34(3):276–9.

40. Gutte H, Hansen AE, Larsen MM, et al. Simultaneous hyperpolarized 13C-Pyruvate MRI and 18F-FDG PET (HyperPET) in 10 dogs with cancer. J Nucl Med 2015;56(11):1786–92.

41. Teixeira SR, Martinez-Rios C, Hu L, et al. Clinical applications of pediatric positron emission tomography-magnetic resonance imaging. Semin Roentgenol 2014;49(4):353–66.

42. Herzog H, Van Den Hoff J. Combined PET/MR systems: an overview and comparison of currently available options. Q J Nucl Med Mol Imaging 2012;56(3): 247–67.

43. Pearce MS, Salotti JA, Little MP, et al. Radiation exposure from CT scans in childhood and subsequent risk of leukaemia and brain tumours: a retrospective cohort study. Lancet 2012;380(9840):499–505.

44. Fahey FH, Treves ST, Adelstein SJ. Minimizing and communicating radiation risk in pediatric nuclear medicine. J Nucl Med 2011;52(8):1240–51.

45. Fahey FH, Treves ST, Adelstein SJ. Minimizing and communicating radiation risk in pediatric nuclear medicine. J Nucl Med Technol 2012;40(1):13–24.

46. Hirsch FW, Sattler B, Sorge I, et al. PET/MR in children. Initial clinical experience in paediatric oncology using an integrated PET/MR scanner. Pediatr Radiol 2013;43(7):860–75.

47. The Scandinavian Sarcoma group guidelines for basic MRI of suspected bone and soft tissue tumours. 2012. Available at: http://www.ssg-org.net/wp-content/uploads/2011/05/Guidelines-for-basic-MRI-examination-of-suspected-bone-and-soft-tissue-tumors.pdf. Accessed March 31, 2016.

48. Aznar MC, Sersar R, Saabye J, et al. Whole-body PET/MRI: the effect of bone attenuation during MR-based attenuation correction in oncology imaging. Eur J Radiol 2014;83(7):1177–83.

49. Ladefoged CN, Hansen AE, Andersen KF, et al. PET/MR imaging of sarcomas: effect of PET quantification by classification of tissue. EJNMMI Phys 2014; 1(Suppl 1):A67.

50. Wagenknecht G, Kaiser HJ, Mottaghy FM, et al. MRI for attenuation correction in PET: methods and challenges. MAGMA 2013;26(1):99–113.

51. Vassiliou V, Andreopoulos D, Frangos S, et al. Bone metastases: assessment of therapeutic response through radiological and nuclear medicine imaging modalities. Clin Oncol 2011;23(9):632–45.

52. Talbot JN, Paycha F, Balogova S. Diagnosis of bone metastasis: recent comparative studies of imaging modalities. Q J Nucl Med Mol Imaging 2011;55(4): 374–410.

53. Yang HL, Liu T, Wang XM, et al. Diagnosis of bone metastases: a meta-analysis comparing (1)(8)FDG PET, CT, MRI and bone scintigraphy. Eur Radiol 2011;21(12):2604–17.

54. Heindel W, Gubitz R, Vieth V, et al. The diagnostic imaging of bone metastases. Dtsch Arztebl Int 2014;111(44):741–7.

55. O'Sullivan GJ, Carty FL, Cronin CG. Imaging of bone metastasis: an update. World J Radiol 2015;7(8): 202–11.

56. Beiderwellen K, Huebner M, Heusch P, et al. Whole-body [(1)(8)F]FDG PET/MRI vs. PET/CT in the assessment of bone lesions in oncological patients: initial results. Eur Radiol 2014;24(8):2023–30.

57. Samarin A, Hullner M, Queiroz MA, et al. 18F-FDG-PET/MR increases diagnostic confidence in detection of bone metastases compared with 18F-FDG-PET/CT. Nucl Med Commun 2015;36(12):1165–73.

58. Spick C, Herrmann K, Czernin J. 18F-FDG PET/CT and PET/MRI perform equally well in cancer: evidence from studies on more than 2,300 patients. J Nucl Med 2016;57(3):420–30.

59. Freitag MT, Radtke JP, Hadaschik BA, et al. Comparison of hybrid (68)Ga-PSMA PET/MRI and (68)Ga-PSMA PET/CT in the evaluation of lymph node and bone metastases of prostate cancer. Eur J Nucl Med Mol Imaging 2016;43(1):70–83.

60. Chaudhari AJ, Bowen SL, Burkett GW, et al. High-resolution (18)F-FDG PET with MRI for monitoring response to treatment in rheumatoid arthritis. Eur J Nucl Med Mol Imaging 2010;37(5):1047.

61. Goerres GW, Forster A, Uebelhart D, et al. F-18 FDG whole-body PET for the assessment of disease activity in patients with rheumatoid arthritis. Clin Nucl Med 2006;31(7):386–90.

62. Palmer WE, Rosenthal DI, Schoenberg OI, et al. Quantification of inflammation in the wrist with gadolinium-enhanced MR imaging and PET with 2-[F-18]-fluoro-2-deoxy-D-glucose. Radiology 1995; 196(3):647–55.

63. Tatsumi M, Yamamoto S, Imaizumi M, et al. Simultaneous PET/MR body imaging in rats: initial experiences with an integrated PET/MRI scanner. Ann Nucl Med 2012;26(5):444–9.

64. Fuchs K, Kohlhofer U, Quintanilla-Martinez L, et al. In vivo imaging of cell proliferation enables the detection of the extent of experimental rheumatoid arthritis by 3'-deoxy-3'-18f-fluorothymidine and small-animal PET. J Nucl Med 2013;54(1):151–8.

PET/MR Imaging in Heart Disease

Christoph Rischpler, MD*, Stephan G. Nekolla, PhD

KEYWORDS

- PET/MR imaging • Heart disease • Cardiac imaging

KEY POINTS

- Hybrid PET/MR imaging is a complex imaging modality that has raised high expectations not only for oncological and neurologic imaging applications but also for cardiac imaging applications.
- Initially, physicians and physicists had to become accustomed to technical challenges, including attenuation correction, gating, and more complex workflow and more elaborate image analysis as compared with PET/computed tomography or standalone MR imaging.
- PET/MR imaging seems to be particularly valuable to assess inflammatory myocardial diseases (such as sarcoidosis), to cross-validate PET versus MR imaging data (eg, myocardial perfusion imaging), and to help validate novel biomarkers of various disease states (eg, postinfarction inflammation).

INTRODUCTION

Approximately 5 to 6 years ago, a new imaging modality entered the clinical market and immediately raised high expectations: integrated PET/MR imaging. Although initial oncological studies were published relatively soon, it took some time until the first cardiac study–related articles were published. The main reason for that may be because integrated cardiac PET/MR imaging is probably among the most complex clinical examinations one can imagine, and physicians and physicists first had to become accustomed to this machine. This review article aims to summarize the reasons for these initial "hormonal difficulties" and tries to shed a light on the most promising and compelling indications for cardiac PET/MR imaging.

TECHNICAL REMARKS REGARDING PET/MR IMAGING IN CARDIOLOGY
General Remarks

High static magnetic fields, rapidly switched gradient fields, and radiofrequency signals disturb conventional photomultiplier tubes and the associated electronics of PET detectors. Furthermore, inferior MR image quality may be the result of electromagnetic interferences and inhomogeneities in a magnetic field through PET detectors. Those were some reasons why building an integrated PET/MR imaging system was deemed for a long time to be a commercially nonviable task to do.

By now, 2 fundamentally different implementations of a PET/MR imaging system are purchasable. One approach was to connect a PET/computed tomography (CT) with a standalone MR imaging system using a table-based common rail system (Philips Ingenuity TF PET/MR imaging [Philips Healthcare, Hamburg, Germany], General Electric (GE) PET/CT-MR imaging [GE Helthcare, Little Chalfont, UK]).[1] The other approach, which allows for (truly) simultaneous imaging, is an integrated PET/MR imaging system (Siemens Biograph mMR [Siemens Healthcare, Erlangen, Germany],[2] GE SIGNA PET/MR imaging[3]). For the truly integrated approach, the aforementioned issues had to be resolved. This was done by using initially avalanche photodiodes (APDs) (ie, photodetectors which are insensitive to magnetic fields

The authors have nothing to disclose.
Department of Nuclear Medicine, Technical University Munich, Ismaninger Straße 22, 81675 München, Germany
* Corresponding author.
E-mail address: C.Rischpler@tum.de

PET Clin 11 (2016) 465–477
http://dx.doi.org/10.1016/j.cpet.2016.05.006
1556-8598/16/$ – see front matter

pet.theclinics.com

even at high field strengths).[4] Siemens eventually used APD-lutetium oxyorthosilicate crystal PET detectors for the Biograph mMR. GE took another path for the SIGNA PET/MR imaging and used silicon photomultiplier technology (SiPM)-based PET detectors that allow, in contrast to the APD technology, time-of-flight PET imaging at less than 400 pico-seconds.[5] By the end of 2010, the first clinical Siemens Biograph mMR worldwide was installed in the department of Nuclear Medicine at the Klinikum Rechts der Isar (Technical University of Munich) as part of a major instrumentation initiative of the German Research Foundation.

Generation of Attenuation Correction Maps from MR Images

Attenuation correction (AC) is an important prerequisite for PET imaging, particularly in cardiac imaging, as non–AC PET images suffer from artifacts and distortion making true quantification and reliable clinical interpretation impossible. Traditionally, AC was performed using either rotating rod sources (eg, Germanium-68 [68Ge]) in standalone PET scanners or making use of the CT component in hybrid PET/CT systems. In integrated PET/MR imaging, these approaches are not feasible; consequently, an alternative method of AC for the 511 keV photons had to be found.

There is no direct physical correlation between MR images and the attenuation caused by the different densities of the imaged tissues. To generate an AC map containing the different attenuation coefficients for 511 keV photons at each voxel within the entire imaged volume is thus a major challenge in PET/MR imaging,[6] particularly as an inaccuracy of the linear attenuation coefficient (μ)-map may substantially degrade cardiac PET images as known from PET/CT.[7] There are different approaches to derive the μ-map from MR images, and the most frequently used ones are based on segmentation, templates, or atlases, or on the PET emission data.

In the segmentation-based method, the AC map is divided into different, disjunct tissue classes to which a certain fixed attenuation coefficient is assigned (this was first proposed by Huang and colleagues[8] in 1981). Based on this concept, our group introduced the idea to use segmented MR-based AC for whole-body PET/MR imaging[9] out of water and fat images generated from a Dixon MR imaging sequence.[10] Usually, this MR imaging sequence requires approximately 18 seconds per bed position to acquire, which is performed during a single breath-hold. Using this method, each voxel may be classified as air or lung, fat, and soft tissue, whereas cortical bone

is virtually impossible to be segmented and is thus ignored (as is in standalone PET devices by the way). Of note, in very sick patients, a breath-hold of 18 seconds may pose a major problem (however, this group of patients is usually not PET/MR imaging–compatible in general). Using an alternative sequence, a T1-weighted turbo spin-echo sequence, a shorter imaging time to generate an AC map is feasible. This, however, happens at the expense of accurate segmentation, as this approach does not allow the differentiation between fat ($\mu = 0.086$ cm^{-1}) and soft tissue ($\mu = 0.096$ cm^{-1}) (on top of not allowing the segmentation of bone).[11] Obviously, the restricted numbers of tissue classes and thus attenuation coefficients is one constraint of the segmentation-based method. In cardiac imaging, this is of considerable importance, as lung tissue is known to show a certain variation regarding morphology and configuration in each patient. Tumor uptake varied between PET/MR imaging and PET/CT in the range of 5% to 15%[9,11] or even up to 23%.[12] Probably because this technique is computationally fast and stable, this approach was implemented (slightly modified) in the first commercially available PET/MR imaging system, the Siemens Biograph mMR.[9] The Philips Ingenuity TF PET/MR imaging also uses a modification of this segmentation-based AC approach.[11] Available data comparing [18F]-2-fluoro-2-deoxy-D-glucose (FDG) uptake between PET/CT and PET/MR imaging reported a high agreement for cardiac imaging,[13,14] and our group also demonstrated a good correlation in oncological studies.[15]

The second AC method is a template-based approach, which tries to match a model to the respective patient's anatomy, in that sense that the known μ-map of the model matches the target. For cranial imaging, a rigid model is obviously sufficient, whereas an elastic registration is a prerequisite for whole-body imaging, making an implementation in daily clinical use complicated. Also, atlas-based approaches are error-prone when variations in anatomy are present (eg, after operations, anatomic variants). To overcome these issues, a combination of template-based and segmentation-based approaches was shown to be feasible for whole-body imaging.[16]

The last approach that needs to be mentioned here is the emission-based method to AC. Here, the PET data itself are used to calculate the μ-map. Photon scatter is one major limitation of this approach.[17] In cardiac imaging, information from emission data was shown to be well-suited for motion correction,[7] and it was also shown to be valuable to recover truncated parts of a μ-map,[18] a common problem in PET/MR imaging particularly in cardiac PET/MR imaging, where parts of the arms are truncated in most scans) as the field of view of the MR imaging is smaller than that of the PET component.

All described methods of AC have advantages and disadvantages; consequently, a combination of the approaches might be most suitable to generate the optimal μ-map, and in the Siemens Biograph mMR, a combined approach was chosen. **Fig. 1** shows the generation of a μ-map and the resulting AC PET images of a patient who was scanned at our institution.

Frequent Issues

MR imaging–related components

In the field of view of the PET component, a multitude of MR imaging–related instruments are present, including the patient bed, positioning aids, and various fixed and variable surface coils. Also, devices such as earphones or, particularly in cardiac imaging, additional monitoring devices (eg, electrocardiogram [ECG], blood pressure cuff, and ventilation belt) and wires are within the field of view of the PET and thus contribute to photon scatter and attenuation. These components may degrade image homogeneity and cause quantification errors, as they are "invisible" for the MR imaging and not incorporated in the μ-map, and will thus not be corrected for in the AC PET images. To minimize these effects, MR imaging components were redesigned by the hardware vendors; however, the attenuation effects are still

detectable, although its unknown if this affects the accuracy of diagnostic scans.[19,20]

Contrast media and foreign bodies

Implantable cardiac devices (eg, implantable cardioverter-defibrillators [ICDs], cardiac resynchronisation therapy [CRT] devices, pacemakers) cause artifacts in CT, which result in an overestimation due to T1-mediated effects of the attenuation and thus in an overestimation of radiotracer uptake in AC PET images, albeit the effect seems not to be relevant.[21] In MR imaging, however, nonmagnetic metallic material results in a signal void exceeding the size of the foreign body, which in turn might cause an underestimation of the attenuation effect and thus ultimately in an overestimation of radiotracer uptake. An even more crucial factor is that such foreign bodies may be heated in an electromagnetic field or become dysfunctional. This leads to one of the major issues in cardiac PET/MR imaging: many patients who have a clinical indication for PET imaging may not even be imaged by PET/MR imaging, and this patient group is increasing.[22,23] Furthermore, the effects of newly developed cardiac devices on PET images are not known (eg, left atrial appendage closure devices, transcatheter aortic heart valves, MicraTM transcatheter pacing system [Medtronic, Dublin, Ireland]). Aside from foreign bodies, MR imaging contrast media may be problematic, as it may cause errors in tissue segmentation because of reduced T1 values.[19] From the authors' own experience, these errors

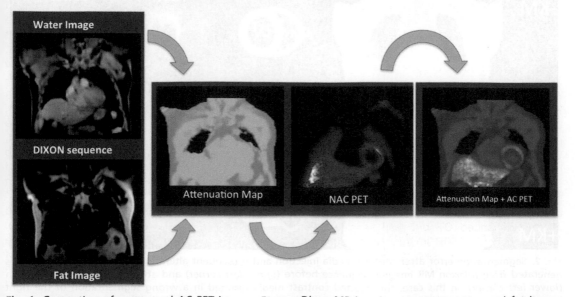

Fig. 1. Generation of μ-map and AC PET images. From a Dixon MR imaging sequence, water and fat images are generated that are used to segment air, lung, fat, and soft tissue. AC PET images are then calculated using this μ-map.

in segmentation frequently occur in the lungs early after contrast administration (**Fig. 2**).

Workflow in Cardiac Imaging

Another important prerequisite for AC is the correct, that is, the most accurate possible, alignment of PET data and μ-map. In PET/CT, different studies have shown that misalignment (caused for example by patient motion) may result in marked artifacts and thus wrong assumptions (eg, inaccurate estimation of regional myocardial blood flow).[7,24] One great advantage of MR imaging over CT is that the AC scan may be repeated as often as needed without any additional radiation to the patient. Multiple μ-maps, however, cause an additional work step, namely, the time-consuming choice of the most accurate μ-map for the acquired PET data. Nevertheless, a satisfactory alignment between PET data and the μ-map can be achieved in most cardiac studies. Of note, most PET studies are acquired over a time range between a few seconds up to 30 minutes or more (depending on the injected radiotracer and the imaging protocol), whereas MR imaging sequences are acquired between 50 ms (per slice in dynamic scans) up to several breath-holds (high-resolution imaging). Therefore, PET imaging time opens a large time window for patient motion (heartbeat, ventilation, body motion), possibly resulting in misaligned PET and MR imaging data. Also, PET data are often acquired nongated (cardiac, respiratory), which then has to be compared with or fused with gated MR imaging data. Last but not least, the acquired PET volume data have to be registered to MR images, which were acquired in multiple (sometimes overlapping) slices in different positions (eg, axial; coronal; sagittal; 2-, 3-, 4-chamber views; short axis). These considerations must be implemented in the imaging protocol/workflow and also in the post-processing work, which is considerably more time-consuming, complex, and error-prone in PET/MR imaging when compared with PET/CT. To mitigate these problems, motion-triggered acquisitions[25] or software corrections,[26] with the aim to enable free-breathing acquisition, are under development.

From the workflow perspective, simultaneous PET/MR imaging is more favorable than sequential PET/MR imaging. The latter is inconvenient for the patient, particularly because it is a lengthy study, whereas it is also inconvenient for the personnel planning the scan, as it is logistically demanding. Therefore, it can be assumed that integrated PET/MR imaging systems increase both patient compliance and patient throughput. However, no data exist regarding whether it is also more cost-efficient than using separate scanners. With regard to cardiac imaging, 3 different potential workflow patterns covering the most-often requested studies (ie, myocardial perfusion, viability, or inflammation) are depicted in **Fig. 3**.

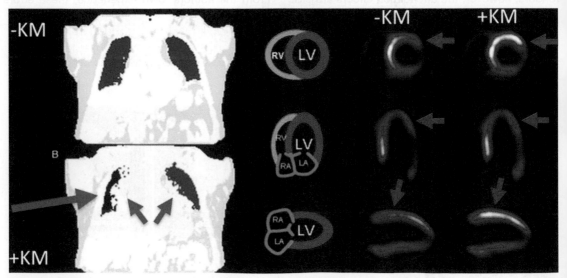

Fig. 2. Segmentation error after contrast media injection and subsequent alteration in AC PET images; μ-maps generated from a Dixon MR imaging sequence before (*upper left corner*) and after contrast media injection (*lower left corner*). In this case, the injected contrast media resulted in a wrong segmentation of the right lung (air instead of lung tissue) and an overestimation of the soft tissue in both hilar regions (*blue arrows*). This in turn caused falsely increased radiotracer uptake (*red arrows*) on the AC PET images in the anterolateral left ventricular myocardial wall. KM, contrast media.

STRESS/REST PERFUSION

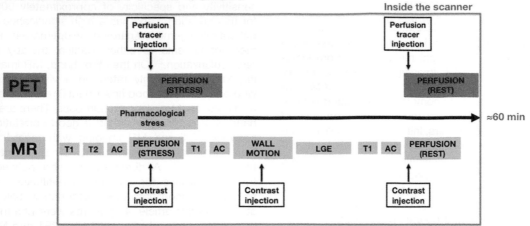

VIABILITY
(including PET perfusion)

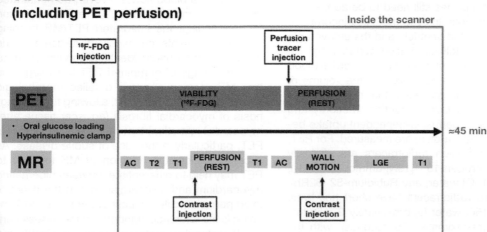

INFLAMMATION
(without PET perfusion)

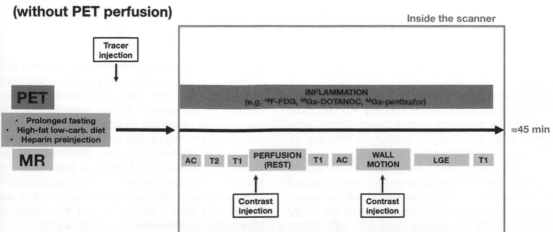

Fig. 3. Potential workflows for cardiac PET/MR imaging studies: (*top*) combined stress/rest perfusion, (*middle*) combined viability and perfusion, (*bottom*) "inflammation protocol."

CLINICAL APPLICATIONS
Myocardial Perfusion Imaging

Myocardial perfusion imaging (MPI) is one of the applications that might really benefit from simultaneous PET/MR imaging acquisition, mainly because of the high in-plane resolution of MR imaging, which could complement the good volume coverage of PET and the superior properties of perfusion radiotracers. Initial studies solely investigated the feasibility of simultaneous PET/MR imaging MPI, and also aimed to cross-validate one modality with the respective other.[27] In addition to that rather technical, research-driven question, a synergistic advantage of simultaneous PET/MR imaging MPI might be the investigation of epicardial versus endocardial blood flow, which might vary in different patient groups (eg, arterial hypertension, diabetes mellitus, kidney failure). In MR imaging, some issues still need to be addressed, which, for example, include the usual incomplete coverage of the left ventricle and the unfavorable properties of gadolinium-based contrast agents. This makes true quantification of myocardial blood flow a very complex task, as only the volume of distribution which excludes the myocytes (ie, effectively only a low "extraction fraction") and not exclusively a perfusion-dependent uptake behavior by the myocardium are measured. For PET, 3 different perfusion radiotracers are clinically available: nitrogen-13 [13N]-ammonia (NH$_3$), oxygen-15 [15O] water, and Rubidium-82 (82Rb). All mentioned radiotracers have short half-lives, particularly 15O water (approximately 2 minutes) and 82Rb (approximately 76 seconds), with the advantage that rest and stress imaging may be performed without lengthy lag times in-between or without the need of background correction.

The unique advantage of simultaneous PET/MR imaging MPI is that both rest and stress perfusion are acquired under completely identical hemodynamic circumstances. Still, one needs to consider that the acquired PET and MR imaging data differ with regard to injection and imaging modes, as the perfusion radiotracer is administered much more slowly than the gadolinium-based contrast agent (PET $\approx$ 30 seconds vs MR imaging $\approx$ 5 seconds) and PET is acquired over a much longer time period than MR imaging (PET $\approx$ 10 minutes vs MR imaging $\approx$ 1 minute).

Besides these mainly technical considerations, now first "real-live" experience has been obtained for the most frequent application in nuclear cardiology: the diagnosis of obstructive coronary artery disease (CAD). On the one hand, PET MPI, which is routinely performed with true quantification of myocardial blood flow, is known to have a

sensitivity and specificity of approximately 90% for this question[28] and has a high significance in patient management regarding the optimal assignment of patients to either medical therapy or revascularization.[29] On the other hand, MR imaging MPI is commonly rated on a visual basis, whereas absolute blood flow quantification is normally reserved for research purposes. There are a handful of reports that found a good correlation between PET and MR imaging with regard to (semi-quantitative) assessment of myocardial blood flow.[30–33] A direct comparison between the 2 modalities for absolute quantification of myocardial blood flow was performed in only 1 study.[34] In this article, 41 patients were pharmacologically stressed and [13N]-NH$_3$ PET and MR imaging values of coronary flow reserve demonstrated a good correlation. The absolute values of myocardial blood flow, however, demonstrated only a rather fair correlation. To reveal the reason for this finding, the integrated PET/MR imaging system represents an excellent device for true cross-validation under identical conditions. Another advantage of combined PET/MR imaging is that MR imaging allows a detailed morphologic characterization of the heart, allowing for the diagnosis of myocardial fibrosis (eg, scar tissue after myocardial infarction) that might be overlooked in PET, particularly in the case of subtle disease. As a consequence, the addition of MR imaging to PET may help to differentiate between hibernating myocardium and myocardial scar in the event of fixed perfusion defects. Last but not least, MR imaging is the reference standard for the assessment of left ventricular function and helps to identify and grade abnormalities in pump function or wall motion. In **Fig. 4**, the simultaneous PET/MR imaging MPI examination of one patient from our institution is depicted.

Myocardial Viability Imaging

"Classic" viability imaging
It is a well-known phenomenon that hypoxia and ischemia cause a shift in myocardial substrate metabolism from free fatty acid oxidation toward glucose consumption. Chronic hypoperfusion or exposure to repetitive stunning lead to a state called "hibernating myocardium," that is, heart tissue that is dysfunctional and demonstrates an increased glucose metabolism, a state that has the potential to be reverted by revascularization.[35] The presence of hibernating myocardium is associated with poor outcome,[36] and the extent of hibernation is of therapeutic significance.[37–39]

Although there are various methods to image myocardial viability (eg, dobutamine stress

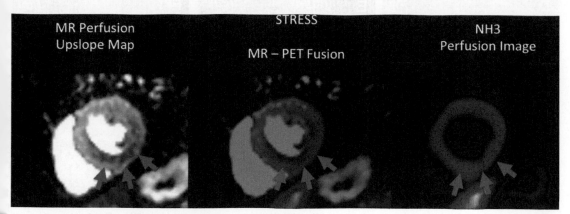

MR Perfusion
Upslope Map

STRESS

MR – PET Fusion

NH3
Perfusion Image

Fig. 4. Simultaneous stress MPI on PET/MR imaging. One representative midventricular short-axis MR image from a simultaneous [13N]-NH₃ PET/MR imaging perfusion study. On the MR upslope map image, an area of subendocardial hypoperfusion (*arrows*) in the inferior wall of the left ventricular myocardium is depicted, which might have been overlooked on PET perfusion images alone.

echocardiography, endocardial ECG-mapping), the most widely used approaches are FDG PET and late gadolinium enhancement (LGE) MR imaging.[40] When using FDG PET, the regional glucose consumption is usually set in relation to the resting myocardial blood flow (assessed for example by [13N]-NH₃ or 82Rb PET). To optimize FDG uptake by cardiomyocytes, which is dependent on the expression of glucose transporters (GLUTs), the patient's metabolic condition is normally standardized by oral glucose loading or by a method called hyperinsulinemic-euglycemic clamping. The sensitivity and specificity of FDG PET for the prediction of regional wall motion recovery after revascularization are approximately 92% and 63%, respectively, based on a meta-analysis.[41] There is increasing evidence that in patients with a significant amount of dysfunctional but viable myocardium, revascularization should be performed without any delay.[42,43]

LGE MR imaging may represent an alternative to FDG PET for viability imaging. In contrast to the PET approach, the proportion of scarred nonviable myocardium is imaged, making use of the fact that gadolinium chelates distribute differently in increased extracellular spaces (ie, fibrotic tissue, such as myocardial scars) and show a reduced washout from these areas in comparison with "healthy" myocardium.[44,45] Despite the opposing approaches of FDG PET and LGE MR imaging (imaging viable vs nonviable tissue), a good correlation between the 2 methods has been demonstrated.[46] Some advantages of LGE MR imaging over FDG PET may be that the kinetics of gadolinium chelates are not dependent on insulin (which might therefore be a valuable alternative in patients with poorly managed diabetes mellitus) and the higher spatial resolution of MR imaging (1–3 mm,

allowing for the differentiation between transmural vs nontransmural scar or between scar and thinned myocardium, for example in heart failure, in the case of reduced FDG uptake).[47] Also, it is known that even small areas of myocardial scar (which may be overlooked on FDG PET) carry prognostic significance in patients with suspicion of CAD but without known myocardial infarction.[48] However, the diagnostic benefit of the combined imaging approach by PET/MR imaging still needs to be shown (**Fig. 5** shows one example of integrated PET/MR imaging viability imaging from our institution). Two studies exist, one from our group and one from the group in Essen, Germany, that compared FDG uptake and the presence of LGE.[49] Both articles describe a substantial agreement between the 2 approaches: it has to be mentioned, however, that imaging was performed shortly after myocardial infarction and not before revascularization, so that the prospective value of hybrid FDG PET/MR imaging regarding wall motion recovery remains unclear.

Postinfarction viability imaging

Our group performed a study using hybrid FDG PET/MR imaging with the aim to compare LGE MR imaging with FDG PET in dysfunctional myocardial segments early after acute myocardial infarction and to evaluate the functional recovery of these segments after 6 months.[50] We found a high intermethod agreement regarding the transmurality of LGE and the decrease of FDG uptake in these segments ($\kappa = 0.65$). Furthermore, the regional wall motion of both the "PET viable" (ie, no or only mild reduction of FDG uptake) and the "MR imaging viable" (nontransmural LGE encompassing <50% of the myocardial segments) dysfunctional segments tended to recover after

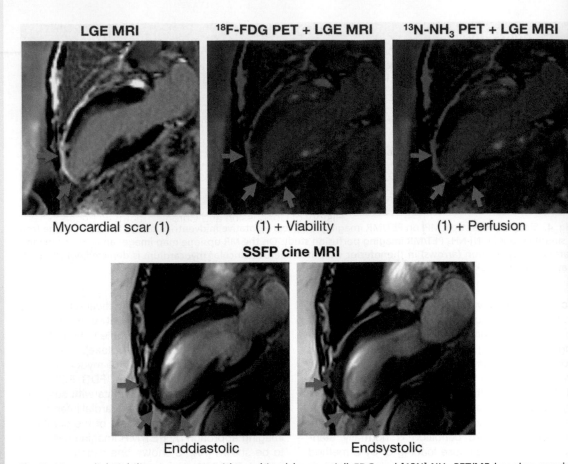

Fig. 5. Myocardial viability assessment with combined (sequential) FDG and [13N]-NH₃ PET/MR imaging acquisition. Blue arrows indicate transmural scar in left ventricular apex (*upper left corner*) with associated absent glucose metabolism (*upper row, middle*), absent perfusion (*upper right corner*), and akinesis (*bottom row*).

6 months. One new and interesting finding in this setting is that there was a small percentage of segments that demonstrated a "discordant" pattern; that is, a downregulated FDG uptake but no or only minor LGE (**Fig. 6**). Interestingly, in only 41% of these "discordant" segments was a functional wall motion improvement observed. However, this was an observational study and the pathologic background of this metabolic alteration of the myocardium remains unclear.

Imaging of Inflammatory Processes in the Myocardium

As described previously, using MR imaging, myocardial fibrosis can be detected with LGE or T1 mapping. Also, MR imaging is the modality of choice to identify myocardial edema, pericardial effusion, or wall motion abnormalities. Taken together, MR imaging is a robust tool to detect processes in the heart that may be associated with inflammatory processes. On the other hand,

an increasing interest in FDG PET for the detection and monitoring of inflammatory processes has occurred over the past few years.[51] The advantage of FDG PET is that it allows estimation of the extent and degree of inflammatory processes, thereby making possible the differentiation between a cured and an ongoing acute inflammatory state. One important prerequisite to be able to use FDG PET for imaging of inflammatory processes in the heart is to switch the myocardium's metabolism from glucose metabolism to fatty acid oxidation. Thereby, the contrast between nonspecific FDG uptake in healthy myocardium on the one hand and in inflammatory processes on the other hand can be dramatically increased. To achieve this, different protocols including prolonged fasting, a low-carbohydrate high-fat diet, or preinjection of heparin before FDG administration have been studied.[52] This nonspecific FDG uptake (particularly in diabetic patients) demonstrates that more specific radiotracers targeting inflammatory

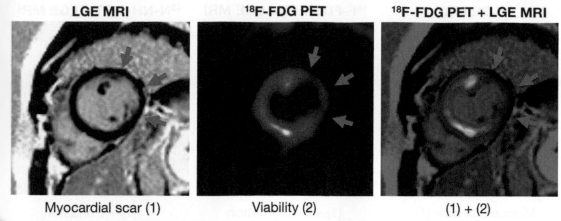

Fig. 6. Alteration of glucose metabolism early after acute myocardial infarction. Early after acute myocardial infarction, a severely reduced glucose metabolism of the lateral left ventricular wall (*blue arrows, middle panel*) is seen on FDG PET, despite only minor myocardial scarring (*blue arrows, left panel*) observed on LGE MR imaging. The right panel demonstrates a fused image of FDG PET and LGE MR imaging (*blue arrows*).

processes are required. One such candidate might be the chemokine receptor 4 ligand Gallium-68 [68Ga] pentixafor.[53]

Myocarditis

Various (primarily viral) infectious diseases, hypersensitivity reactions, or autoimmune diseases may be the cause of myocarditis. Although MR imaging is increasingly used to guarantee the diagnosis, the reference standard is still endomyocardial biopsy. The infiltrative changes in the myocardium, which typically take place in the epicardium of the free wall, may be depicted by gadolinium-enhanced double-inversion-recovery fast spin-echo T2-weighted and T1-weighted sequences or also LGE MR imaging.[54]

Just recently, the interest to use FDG PET to diagnose, grade, and monitor myocarditis seems to have increased, and there are some initial publications describing a successful application in this clinical setting, particularly in inconclusive cases.[55–57] Also, FDG PET may represent an alternative in patients who are not compatible with MR imaging. Whether or not the combined approach of FDG PET/MR imaging results in an improved diagnosis and patient management needs to be further studied.

Sarcoidosis

Cardiac involvement by sarcoidosis is a dangerous manifestation, as the initial clinical "presentation" is sudden cardiac death in up to 40% of cases.[58] This disease is typically characterized by an infiltration of inflammatory granulomas, eventually resulting in postinflammatory scars, which in turn may cause conduction abnormalities, arrythmias, and heart failure. This

illustrates the reason that cardiac involvement by sarcoidosis needs to be excluded. The worldwide standard for the diagnosis are the guidelines of the Japanese Ministry of Health and Welfare; these guidelines recommend the application of MR imaging or Gallium-67 (67Ga) scintigraphy. FDG PET, however, is not implemented in these guidelines, even though there is accumulating evidence demonstrating that FDG PET may be valuable for initial diagnosis, monitoring, and therapeutic guidance. As such, more recent expert consensus guidelines recommend the application of this modality.[59] In addition to FDG PET, it also may be valuable to investigate myocardial perfusion (eg, [13N]-NH₃ PET), as this combined approach allows for the differentiation between active acute inflammation (normal perfusion, intense FDG uptake), advanced stages of cardiac involvement (reduced perfusion, intense FDG uptake) (**Fig. 7**), or end-stage disease (reduced or absent perfusion, absent FDG uptake).[60] In combination with MR imaging, the exact illustration of fibrotic tissue using LGE might be valuable for exact lead placement in the event of ICD implantation.[61]

Imaging postinfarction inflammation with PET/MR imaging

After myocardial infarction, the postischemic myocardium undergoes a complex healing process, which involves a vivid inflammatory process. This inflammatory reaction just recently came into the focus of cardiac research. Recent publications indicate that an intense inflammation in the heart after myocardial infarction may result in adverse remodeling and adverse outcome, similar to established prognostic markers such as infarct

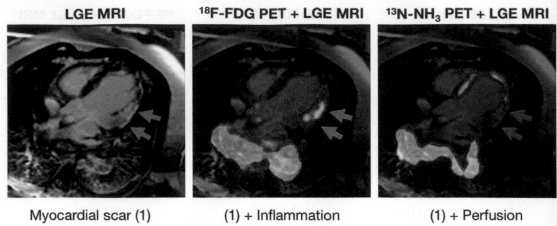

Fig. 7. PET/MR imaging in a patient with cardiac sarcoidosis. On LGE MR image, scarring of the basal lateral wall of the left ventricle can be seen (*blue arrows, left panel*). On PET images, intense FDG uptake reflecting increased glucose metabolism (*yellow arrows, middle panel*) and severely reduced myocardial perfusion (*red arrows, right panel*) in the same region are observed, indicating an advanced stage of cardiac involvement by sarcoidosis. Intense FDG uptake in hilar and mediastinal lymph nodes is another very common manifestation of sarcoidosis, which is also visualized (*middle panel*).

size or postinfarction ejection fraction.[62] Monocytes, which can be subcharacterized based on certain surface markers into classic, nonclassic, and intermediate populations, are thought to play a pivotal role in this complex inflammatory reaction. Recently, Nahrendorf and colleagues demonstrated that this monocyte-driven inflammatory process in the heart may be imaged in rodents using FDG PET/MR imaging,[63] and it was subsequently shown that this imaging strategy can be translated into humans.[64] In a very recently published article, our group demonstrated that the intensity of postischemic FDG uptake in the heart is

a prognostic marker for the functional recovery of the left ventricle independent of infarct size (**Fig. 8**).[65] Based on these findings, FDG PET/MR imaging may be an ideal tool to monitor the effects of novel interventions modulating this inflammatory reaction.

SUMMARY

The onset of hybrid PET/MR imaging scanners raised high expectations not only for oncological and neurologic imaging applications but also for cardiac imaging applications. Early after the first

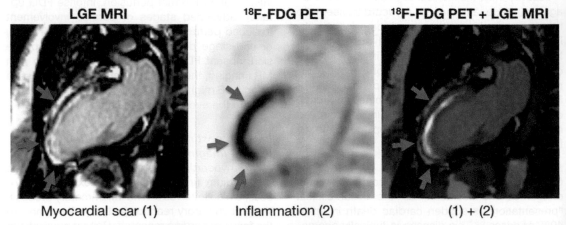

Fig. 8. Postischemic myocardial inflammation after acute ST-elevation myocardial infarction. FDG PET/MR imaging 2-chamber views of a patient early after acute myocardial infarction reveals mostly transmural myocardial LGE (*blue arrows, left panel*) on MR imaging with corresponding intense glucose metabolism (*blue arrows, middle panel*) on PET as a sign of postischemic myocardial inflammation. The fused 2-chamber view demonstrates colocalization of myocardial scarring and inflammatory reaction (*blue arrows, right panel*).

tomographs entered the market, physicians and physicists had to deal with technical challenges, such as AC, gating, and more complex workflows and more elaborate image analysis as compared with PET/CT or standalone MR imaging. Now, increasing numbers of publications with a focus on cardiac imaging are emerging, and the additional value of combined PET/MR imaging is becoming clear: cardiac diseases can now be imaged morphologically as well as functionally and molecularly to most optimally reveal the underlying causes or acuity of disease. In addition, PET/MR imaging represents an ideal research platform to compare various pathophysiological components of disease (eg, myocardial perfusion, viability) or to validate novel biomarkers of various disease states (eg, postinfarction inflammation). However, future studies will have to determine whether integrated PET/MR imaging will become routine in clinical use or even become irreplaceable for certain clinical indications.

REFERENCES

1. Zaidi H, Ojha N, Morich M, et al. Design and performance evaluation of a whole-body Ingenuity TF PET-MRI system. Phys Med Biol 2011;56(10):3091–106.

2. Delso G, Furst S, Jakoby B, et al. Performance measurements of the Siemens mMR integrated whole-body PET/MR scanner. J Nucl Med 2011;52(12):1914–22.

3. Levin CS, Maramraju SH, Khalighi MM, et al. Design features and mutual compatibility studies of the time-of-flight PET capable GE SIGNA PET/MR system. IEEE Trans Med Imaging 2016. [Epub ahead of print].

4. Pichler BJ, Judenhofer MS, Catana C, et al. Performance test of an LSO-APD detector in a 7-T MRI scanner for simultaneous PET/MRI. J Nucl Med 2006;47(4):639–47.

5. Levin C, Deller T, Peterson W, et al. Initial results of simultaneous whole-body ToF PET/MR. J Nucl Med 2014;55(Suppl 1):660.

6. Hofmann M, Pichler B, Scholkopf B, et al. Towards quantitative PET/MRI: a review of MR-based attenuation correction techniques. Eur J Nucl Med Mol Imaging 2009;36(Suppl 1):S93–104.

7. Martinez-Moller A, Souvatzoglou M, Navab N, et al. Artifacts from misaligned CT in cardiac perfusion PET/CT studies: frequency, effects, and potential solutions. J Nucl Med 2007;48(2):188–93.

8. Huang SC, Carson RE, Phelps ME, et al. A boundary method for attenuation correction in positron computed tomography. J Nucl Med 1981;22(7):627–37.

9. Martinez-Moller A, Souvatzoglou M, Delso G, et al. Tissue classification as a potential approach for attenuation correction in whole-body PET/MRI: evaluation with PET/CT data. J Nucl Med 2009;50(4):520–6.

10. Coombs BD, Szumowski J, Coshow W. Two-point Dixon technique for water-fat signal decomposition with B0 inhomogeneity correction. Magn Reson Med 1997;38(6):884–9.

11. Schulz V, Torres-Espallardo I, Renisch S, et al. Automatic, three-segment, MR-based attenuation correction for whole-body PET/MR data. Eur J Nucl Med Mol Imaging 2011;38(1):138–52.

12. Samarin A, Burger C, Wollenweber SD, et al. PET/MR imaging of bone lesions–implications for PET quantification from imperfect attenuation correction. Eur J Nucl Med Mol Imaging 2012;39(7):1154–60.

13. Lau MCJ, Laforest R, Sotoudeh H, et al. Evaluation of attenuation correction in cardiac PET using PET/MR. Circulation 2014;130:A17980.

14. Nekolla SG, Cabello J. The foundation layer of quantitative cardiac PET/MRI: attenuation correction. Again. J Nucl Cardiol 2016. [Epub ahead of print].

15. Drzezga A, Souvatzoglou M, Eiber M, et al. First clinical experience with integrated whole-body PET/MR: comparison to PET/CT in patients with oncologic diagnoses. J Nucl Med 2012;53(6):845–55.

16. Hofmann M, Bezrukov I, Mantlik F, et al. MRI-based attenuation correction for whole-body PET/MRI: quantitative evaluation of segmentation- and atlas-based methods. J Nucl Med 2011;52(9):1392–9.

17. Nuyts J, Dupont P, Stroobants S, et al. Simultaneous maximum a posteriori reconstruction of attenuation and activity distributions from emission sinograms. IEEE Trans Med Imaging 1999;18(5):393–403.

18. Nuyts J, Bal G, Kehren F, et al. Completion of a truncated attenuation image from the attenuated PET emission data. IEEE Trans Med Imaging 2013;32(2):237–46.

19. Fürst S, Souvatzoglu M, Rischpler C, et al. Effects of MR contrast agents on attenuation map generation and cardiac PET quantification in PET/MR. J Nucl Med 2012;53(Suppl 1):139.

20. MacDonald LR, Kohlmyer S, Liu C, et al. Effects of MR surface coils on PET quantification. Med Phys 2011;38(6):2948–56.

21. DiFilippo FP, Brunken RC. Do implanted pacemaker leads and ICD leads cause metal-related artifact in cardiac PET/CT? J Nucl Med 2005;46(3):436–43.

22. Marinskis G, Bongiorni MG, Dagres N, et al. Performing magnetic resonance imaging in patients with implantable pacemakers and defibrillators: results of a European Heart Rhythm Association survey. Europace 2012;14(12):1807–9.

23. Cohen JD, Costa HS, Russo RJ. Determining the risks of magnetic resonance imaging at 1.5 tesla for patients with pacemakers and implantable cardioverter defibrillators. Am J Cardiol 2012;110(11):1631–6.

24. Gould KL, Pan T, Loghin C, et al. Frequent diagnostic errors in cardiac PET/CT due to misregistration of CT attenuation and emission PET images: a definitive analysis of causes, consequences, and corrections. J Nucl Med 2007;48(7):1112–21.

25. Adluru G, Chen L, Kim SE, et al. Three-dimensional late gadolinium enhancement imaging of the left atrium with a hybrid radial acquisition and compressed sensing. J Magn Reson Imaging 2011; 34(6):1465–71.

26. Xue H, Zuehlsdorff S, Kellman P, et al. Unsupervised inline analysis of cardiac perfusion MRI. Med Image Comput Comput Assist Interv 2009; 12(Pt 2):741–9.

27. Zhang HS, Rischpler C, Souvatzoglou M, et al. First simultaneous measurement of myocardial perfusion on whole-body PET/MR. J Nucl Med 2012;53(Suppl 1):29.

28. Parker MW, Iskandar A, Limone B, et al. Diagnostic accuracy of cardiac positron emission tomography versus single photon emission computed tomography for coronary artery disease a bivariate meta-analysis. Circ Cardiovasc Imaging 2012;5(6):700–7.

29. Hachamovitch R, Hayes SW, Friedman JD, et al. Comparison of the short-term survival benefit associated with revascularization compared with medical therapy in patients with no prior coronary artery disease undergoing stress myocardial perfusion single photon emission computed tomography. Circulation 2003;107(23):2900–7.

30. Schwitter J, Nanz D, Kneifel S, et al. Assessment of myocardial perfusion in coronary artery disease by magnetic resonance—a comparison with positron emission tomography and coronary angiography. Circulation 2001;103(18):2230–5.

31. Ibrahim T, Nekolla SG, Schreiber K, et al. Assessment of coronary flow reserve: comparison between contrast-enhanced magnetic resonance imaging and positron emission tomography. J Am Coll Cardiol 2002;39(5):864–70.

32. Parkka JP, Niemi P, Saraste A, et al. Comparison of MRI and positron emission tomography for measuring myocardial perfusion reserve in healthy humans. Magn Reson Med 2006;55(4):772–9.

33. Fritz-Hansen T, Hove JD, Kofoed KF, et al. Quantification of MRI measured myocardial perfusion reserve in healthy humans: a comparison with positron emission tomography. J Magn Reson Imaging 2008;27(4):818–24.

34. Morton G, Chiribiri A, Ishida M, et al. Quantification of absolute myocardial perfusion in patients with coronary artery disease: comparison between cardiac magnetic resonance and positron emission tomography. J Am Coll Cardiol 2012;60(16):1546–55.

35. Heyndrickx GR, Millard RW, McRitchie RJ, et al. Regional myocardial functional and electrophysiological alterations after brief coronary artery occlusion in conscious dogs. J Clin Invest 1975; 56(4):978–85.

36. Beanlands RS, Hendry PJ, Masters RG, et al. Delay in revascularization is associated with increased mortality rate in patients with severe left ventricular dysfunction and viable myocardium on fluorine 18-fluorodeoxyglucose positron emission tomography imaging. Circulation 1998;98(19 Suppl):II51–6.

37. Di Carli MF, Davidson M, Little R, et al. Value of metabolic imaging with positron emission tomography for evaluating prognosis in patients with coronary artery disease and left ventricular dysfunction. Am J Cardiol 1994;73(8):527–33.

38. D'Egidio G, Nichol G, Williams KA, et al. Increasing benefit from revascularization is associated with increasing amounts of myocardial hibernation: a substudy of the PARR-2 trial. JACC Cardiovasc Imaging 2009;2(9):1060–8.

39. Allman KC, Shaw LJ, Hachamovitch R, et al. Myocardial viability testing and impact of revascularization on prognosis in patients with coronary artery disease and left ventricular dysfunction: a meta-analysis. J Am Coll Cardiol 2002;39(7):1151–8.

40. Tillisch J, Brunken R, Marshall R, et al. Reversibility of cardiac wall-motion abnormalities predicted by positron tomography. N Engl J Med 1986;314(14): 884–8.

41. Schinkel AF, Poldermans D, Elhendy A, et al. Assessment of myocardial viability in patients with heart failure. J Nucl Med 2007;48(7):1135–46.

42. Bax JJ, Schinkel AF, Boersma E, et al. Early versus delayed revascularization in patients with ischemic cardiomyopathy and substantial viability: impact on outcome. Circulation 2003;108(Suppl 1):II39–42.

43. Beanlands RS, Ruddy TD, deKemp RA, et al. Positron emission tomography and recovery following revascularization (PARR-1): the importance of scar and the development of a prediction rule for the degree of recovery of left ventricular function. J Am Coll Cardiol 2002;40(10):1735–43.

44. Klein C, Nekolla SG, Balbach T, et al. The influence of myocardial blood flow and volume of distribution on late Gd-DTPA kinetics in ischemic heart failure. J Magn Reson Imaging 2004;20(4):588–93.

45. Klein C, Schmal TR, Nekolla SG, et al. Mechanism of late gadolinium enhancement in patients with acute myocardial infarction. J Cardiovasc Magn Reson 2007;9(4):653–8.

46. Klein C, Nekolla SG, Bengel FM, et al. Assessment of myocardial viability with contrast-enhanced magnetic resonance imaging: comparison with positron emission tomography. Circulation 2002;105(2):162–7.

47. Kim RJ, Wu E, Rafael A, et al. The use of contrast-enhanced magnetic resonance imaging to identify reversible myocardial dysfunction. N Engl J Med 2000;343(20):1445–53.

48. Kwong RY, Chan AK, Brown KA, et al. Impact of un-recognized myocardial scar detected by cardiac magnetic resonance imaging on event-free survival in patients presenting with signs or symptoms of coronary artery disease. Circulation 2006;113(23): 2733–43.

49. Nensa F, Poeppel TD, Beiderwellen K, et al. Hybrid PET/MR imaging of the heart: feasibility and initial results. Radiology 2013;268(2):366–73.

50. Rischpler C, Langwieser N, Souvatzoglou M, et al. PET/MRI early after myocardial infarction: evaluation of viability with late gadolinium enhancement transmurality vs. 18F-FDG uptake. Eur Heart J Cardiovasc Imaging 2015;16(6):661–9.

51. Erba PA, Sollini M, Lazzeri E, et al. FDG-PET in cardiac infections. Semin Nucl Med 2013;43(5):377–95.

52. Scholtens AM, Verberne HJ, Budde RP, et al. Additional heparin preadministration improves cardiac glucose metabolism suppression over low-carbohydrate diet alone in 18F-FDG PET imaging. J Nucl Med 2016;57(4):568–73.

53. Rischpler C, Nekolla SG, Kossmann H, et al. Upregulated myocardial CXCR4-expression after myocardial infarction assessed by simultaneous GA-68 pentixafor PET/MRI. J Nucl Cardiol 2016; 23(1):131–3.

54. Sparrow PJ, Merchant N, Provost YL, et al. CT and MR imaging findings in patients with acquired heart disease at risk for sudden cardiac death. Radiographics 2009;29(3):805–23.

55. Nensa F, Poeppel TD, Krings P, et al. Multiparametric assessment of myocarditis using simultaneous positron emission tomography/magnetic resonance imaging. Eur Heart J 2014;35(32):2173.

56. von Olshausen G, Hyafil F, Langwieser N, et al. Detection of acute inflammatory myocarditis in Epstein Barr virus infection using hybrid 18F-fluoro-deoxyglucose-positron emission tomography/magnetic resonance imaging. Circulation 2014;130(11):925–6.

57. Piriou N, Sassier J, Pallardy A, et al. Utility of cardiac FDG-PET imaging coupled to magnetic resonance for the management of an acute myocarditis with non-informative endomyocardial biopsy. Eur Heart J Cardiovasc Imaging 2015;16(5):574.

58. Sekiguchi M, Numao Y, Imai M, et al. Clinical and histopathological profile of sarcoidosis of the heart and acute idiopathic myocarditis. Concepts through a study employing endomyocardial biopsy. I. Sarcoidosis. Jpn Circ J 1980;44(4):249–63.

59. Birnie DH, Sauer WH, Bogun F, et al. HRS expert consensus statement on the diagnosis and management of arrhythmias associated with cardiac sarcoidosis. Heart Rhythm 2014;11(7):1305–23.

60. Blankstein R, Osborne M, Naya M, et al. Cardiac positron emission tomography enhances prognostic assessments of patients with suspected cardiac sarcoidosis. J Am Coll Cardiol 2014;63(4):329–36.

61. Schneider S, Batrice A, Rischpler C, et al. Utility of multimodal cardiac imaging with PET/MRI in cardiac sarcoidosis: implications for diagnosis, monitoring and treatment. Eur Heart J 2014;35(5):312.

62. van der Laan AM, Nahrendorf M, Piek JJ. Healing and adverse remodelling after acute myocardial infarction: role of the cellular immune response. Heart 2012;98(18):1384–90.

63. Lee WW, Marinelli B, van der Laan AM, et al. PET/MRI of inflammation in myocardial infarction. J Am Coll Cardiol 2012;59(2):153–63.

64. Wollenweber T, Roentgen P, Schafer A, et al. Characterizing the inflammatory tissue response to acute myocardial infarction by clinical multimodality noninvasive imaging. Circ Cardiovasc Imaging 2014;7(5): 811–8.

65. Rischpler C, Dirschinger RJ, Nekolla SG, et al. Prospective evaluation of 18F-fluorodeoxyglucose uptake in postischemic myocardium by simultaneous positron emission tomography/magnetic resonance imaging as a prognostic marker of functional outcome. Circ Cardiovasc Imaging 2016;9(4):e004316.

PET/MR Imaging in Vascular Disease
Atherosclerosis and Inflammation

Rasmus Sejersten Ripa, MD, DMSc,
Sune Folke Pedersen, PhD, Andreas Kjær, MD, PhD, DMSc*

KEYWORDS

- PET/MR • PET/CT • Molecular imaging • Atherosclerosis • Vulnerable plaque
- Cardiovascular disease • Inflammation • Macrophages

KEY POINTS

- For evaluation of risk of thromboembolic events, such as stroke and acute myocardial infarction, molecular imaging of plaque vulnerability is more relevant than the degree of stenosis.
- PET/MR imaging is a favorable combination for plaque imaging, as PET can visualize plaque activity and MR imaging can visualize plaque composition.
- Vascular imaging of atherosclerosis and atherosclerotic plaques may become a major application of hybrid PET/MR imaging.
- So far, surprisingly few studies using PET/MR imaging for imaging of atherosclerosis have been published.

INTRODUCTION

Within imaging of atherosclerotic disease, in everyday clinical practice the approach of lumenography using computed tomography (CT), ultrasonography, or invasive angiography is still the backbone of evaluation. Although this approach has merit as preoperative evaluation, that is, whether invasive procedures, such as endarterectomy, percutaneous coronary intervention, and coronary artery bypass grafting, to remove stenosis are likely to be successful, these methods are less effective to predict the likelihood of future thromboembolic events caused by vulnerability of plaques. As an example of the shortcoming of using the degree of stenosis for risk stratification is the selection of patients that shall undergo carotid endarterectomy. Here the numbers needed to treat are as high as 6 to 1.[1] Accordingly, it is increasingly acknowledged that molecular and functional imaging approaches are needed. Both PET and MR imaging have been used separately for plaque characterization, whereas this is not to the same extent the case for CT, apart from evaluation of calcification; therefore, the use of hybrid imaging with PET/MR imaging may seem particularly relevant for the evaluation of atherosclerosis and plaques. Indeed, at the fourth International Workshop on PET/MR Imaging held in Tübingen in 2015 there was in particular optimism for the use of PET/MR imaging in cardiovascular disease where it was even suggested that it could become a primary clinical application of hybrid PET/MR imaging.[2] Here, the authors shall not judge whether

The authors have nothing to disclose. The authors have received generous support from the John & Birthe Meyer Foundation, the National Advanced Technology Foundation, The Innovation Fund Denmark, Danish Medical Research Council, Rigshospitalet Research Foundation, Svend Andersen Foundation, AP Møller Foundation, Novo Nordisk Foundation, and Lundbeck Foundation to perform studies reported here.
Department of Clinical Physiology, Nuclear Medicine & PET and Cluster for Molecular Imaging, Rigshospitalet and University of Copenhagen, KF-4012, Rigshosptialet, Blegdamsvej 9, Copenhagen 2100, Denmark
* Corresponding author.
E-mail address: akjaer@sund.ku.dk

PET Clin 11 (2016) 479–488
http://dx.doi.org/10.1016/j.cpet.2016.05.009
1556-8598/16/$ – see front matter © 2016 Elsevier Inc. All rights reserved.

this is the case. However, later the authors go through some of the possibilities and arguments for the use of PET/MR imaging in atherosclerotic imaging in patients that could support the optimism put forward.

MR IMAGING FOR PLAQUE CHARACTERIZATION

Whereas MR imaging can also be used for luminal angiography as can CT, it is of more interest that magnetic resonance (MR) is capable of characterizing the atherosclerotic plaques with respect to key components linked to risk of vulnerability.[3] First, MR does visualize the vessel wall and can, therefore, be used to quantify the volumetric plaque burden. This can also be used to follow changes in plaque burden following therapeutic interventions. Currently, 2-dimensional plaque thickness is most often used but 3-dimensional volumetric measurement is possible. For risk assessment and identification of high-risk plaques more likely to lead to thromboembolic events, such as as stroke and myocardial infarction, several key features of the vulnerable plaque may be visualized with MR. These features include a large necrotic core, demonstration of remodeling, intraplaque hemorrhage and presence of a thin fibrous cap of the plaque. For each of these characteristics, MR imaging is probably the method of choice. Development of fast MR sequences optimal for the different characteristics is currently a key area for vascular MR research. In general, it should be noted that for any imaging modality visualization of vessels like the carotid arteries is less challenging than for the coronary arteries. Accordingly, not all the mentioned capabilities, including the PET tracers described later, may be applicable at this point for the coronaries. However, when it is possible to use for carotid imaging and demonstrating value here, the authors think the technical challenges to move into coronary imaging is likely to be overcome in the future.

MR is also capable of demonstrating angiogenesis and inflammation. For angiogenesis, dynamic gadolinium enhancement has been shown to correlate with evidence of plaque angiogenesis.[4] For visualization of plaque inflammation, ultrasmall superparamagnetic particles of iron oxide (USPIO) have been used with success.[5,6] The method is based on uptake of USPIO by activated macrophages leading to an increased concentration in active, vulnerable plaques. However, in a context of PET/MR hybrid imaging it should be noted that both angiogenesis as well as inflammation may also be imaged with more specific PET tracers and with higher sensitivity (see later discussion).

PET FOR MOLECULAR IMAGING OF PLAQUE DEVELOPMENT AND VULNERABILITY

For clinical use, there is currently probably no better noninvasive imaging method than PET for following the molecular events in the development of atherosclerotic plaques and monitoring when they become vulnerable. The biology of plaque development is increasingly well understood at the cellular and molecular level. A review of this[7] is clearly beyond the scope of the current article, but it can be roughly summarized as follows. The initial pathology is endothelia dysfunction with decreased bioavailability of nitric oxide. Subsequently, a proinflammatory state results with expression of vascular and intercellular adhesion molecules, such as vascular cell adhesion molecule-1 (VCAM-1) and intercellular adhesion molecule-1 (ICAM-1), by the endothelial cells that lead to monocyte recruitment. Monocytes that infiltrate the arterial intima then differentiate into macrophages that in turn engulf lipids, in particular oxidized low-density lipoproteins resulting in macrophages transforming into foam cells and leading to the macroscopically observable fatty streaks on the vessel wall. When this process advances, a necrotic core is formed and further influx of leucocytes is stimulated leading to a thrombogenic core. At this point vascular smooth muscle cells migrate into the lesion and, by modifications of extracellular matrix, lead to formation of a fibrous cap on the luminal part of the plaque. In parallel, hypoxia in the plaque stimulates angiogenesis with formation of immature vessel sprouting from the *vasa vasorum* causing plaque hemorrhage and further recruitment of leucocytes. Further events, taking place during development of the plaque, are foam cells becoming apoptotic as well as microcalcification of the plaque. At the end stage, the plaque is metabolically active and covered by a thin fibrous cap, which may easily rupture.

From a PET imaging point of view, it is of interest that there exist PET tracers targeting almost any of the molecular events in plaque formation[8] (**Fig. 1**). On the preclinical level several studies have been undertaken on how different PET tracers reflect the development of atherosclerosis and (vulnerable) plaque.[9] In the current review, the authors focus only on clinical studies undertaken so far. As with other areas of PET imaging, we can divide research into use of fluorodeoxyglucose (FDG) and non-FDG tracers.

18F-fluorodeoxyglucose-PET for Atherosclerosis and Plaque Imaging

For FDG-PET the bulk of work has been on how FDG uptake in the arterial wall correlates with cardiovascular risk and plaque features. The first

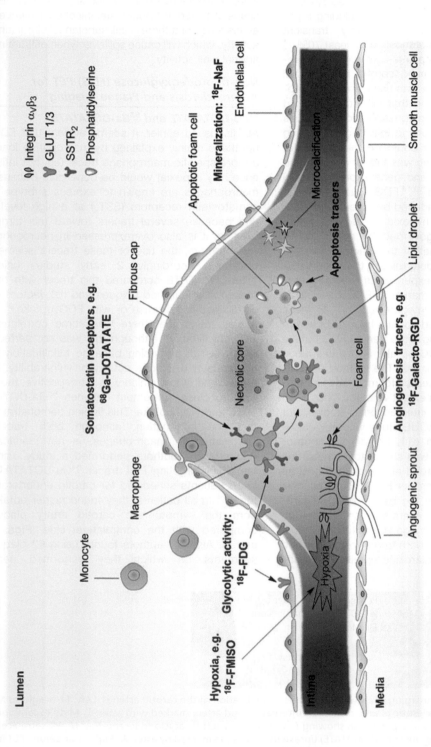

Fig. 1. Atherosclerosis and molecular imaging: the vulnerable atherosclerotic plaque protrudes into the vessel lumen as a result of progressive inflammation of the vessel wall intima. Monocytes are continuously recruited from the blood and into the intima where they differentiate to macrophages and become foam cells due to lipid ingestion. Eventually foam cells are overcome and become apoptotic amassing to a lipid-rich necrotic core, which is covered by a thin fibrous cap. Expansion of the intima leads to hypoxia, which drives angiogenesis whereby new blood vessels sprout from the *vasa vasorum* in the vessel wall media. PET tracers are depicted in blue, and arrows point to their respective molecular targets. ^{18}F-FDG, 2-(^{18}F)-fluoro-2-deoxy-D-glucose; ^{18}F-FMISO, ^{18}F-fluoromisonidazole; ^{18}F-NaF, ^{18}F-sodium fluoride; ^{68}Ga-DOTA-TATE, ^{68}Ga-(1,4,7,10-tetraazacyclododecane-N,N',N'',N'''-tetra-acetic acid)-d-Phe^1,Tyr^3-octreotate; GLUT, glucose transporter; Integrin $\alpha_v\beta_3$, integrin receptor dimer al-pha$_v$beta$_3$; SSTR$_2$, somatostatin receptor subtype 2. (*From* Pedersen SF, Hag AMF, Klausen TL, et al. Positron emission tomography of the vulnerable atherosclerotic plaque in man–a contemporary review. Clin Physiol Funct Imaging 2014;34(6):417; with permission.)

report on vascular uptake of FDG came in 2001 and was retrospective.[10] It demonstrated increasing uptake with age. This report was followed by a prospective study the following year including 8 patients with recent carotid-territory transient ischemic attack and a stenosis of at least 70%.[11] In 6 patients, contralateral lesions were also present at the asymptomatic carotid artery. In all cases, the FDG uptake was highest at the symptomatic lesion indicating that FDG uptake could indicate vulnerability of plaques. Removed plaques showed heavy macrophage infiltration indicating that macrophage load could be the reason for FDG avidity. This finding was further documented both at the protein[12] and gene expression level using CD68 as a target.[13,14] FDG visualized glycolysis, which in turn is induced by several molecular processes, including hypoxia.[15] Also PET tracer availability may be governed by perfusion. To further investigate whether the macrophage load was indeed the major determinant, the authors performed a series of experiments whereby they looked into hypoxia marker HIF-1α as well as angiogenesis marker integrin $\alpha_V\beta_3$.[16,17] In these studies, the authors did not find hypoxia or angiogenesis to be a driving force behind FDG uptake further supporting FDG uptake in plaques being governed by macrophages. The method of FDG-PET has now been accepted for monitoring atherosclerotic activity to an extent whereby it has been included in several interventional studies, for example, the dal-PLAQUE study whereby dalcetrapib in combination with low-density lipoprotein–lowering therapy was shown to decrease the FDG uptake in the carotid arteries.[18] It should be noted that using the proper FDG-PET protocol is essential for obtaining the best results. Accordingly, the authors and others have shown that the optimal time point for image acquisition is 3 hours after injection and that both target-to-background ratios as well as standardized uptake value may

be used.[19,20] Confusion was present in the early days of research in this area, as many studies were retrospective reusing oncological FDG-PET scans obtained at 1 hours after injection. However at this time point there is still substantial circulating activity, which will cause spillover when estimating arterial wall activity.

Non-fluorodeoxyglucose (FDG)-PET for Atherosclerosis and Plaque Imaging

^{64}Cu-DOTATATE and ^{68}Ga-DOTATATE

As discussed earlier, it seems evident that FDG uptake is mainly explained by macrophage load; a more specific macrophage tracer (eg, not influenced by hypoxia) would be beneficial. Because macrophages are known to express subtype 2 somatostatin receptors (SST_2) at a high level[21] and because several tracers toward this target exist as it is also overexpressed in neuroendocrine tumors, the use of these tracers seemed obvious. Accordingly, 2 early studies using ^{68}Ga-DOTATATE compared this tracer with the presence of calcified plaques and risk factors of cardiovascular disease or with FDG uptake.[22,23] It was found that there was some correlation with calcification, although this was not perfect, which is not surprising because calcification is no indicator of plaque activity or vulnerability. In the second study, which was retrospective, there was no close agreement between ^{68}Ga-DOTATATE and FDG uptake. This finding demonstrates that the information, although both tracers are related to macrophages, is not identical. Recently, the authors performed a study using the SST_2 targeting PET tracer ^{64}Cu-DOTATATE in 10 patients scheduled for carotid endarterectomy.[24] In all patients, they found higher uptake from the symptomatic carotid artery plaque compared with the contralateral side (**Figs. 2** and **3**). Also the authors found, using 62 plaque segments on which they performed gene

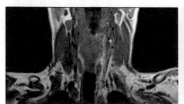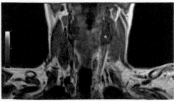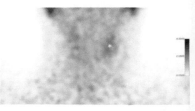

Fig. 2. Coronal PET/MR imaging of the neck region for visualization of the carotid arteries. Left: T1-weighted MR image showing atherosclerotic plaque of the left internal carotid artery marked with asterisk. Middle: combined PET/MR imaging of the same projection showing (^{64}Cu) (1,4,7,10-tetraazacyclododecane-*N*,*N'*,*N''*,*N'''*-tetra-acetic acid)-*d*-Phe1,Tyr3-octreotate (^{64}Cu-DOTATATE) uptake in the plaque marked by asterisk. Right: standalone PET image of the same projection showing ^{64}Cu-DOTATATE distribution and left carotid artery plaque marked by asterisk. (*From* Pedersen SF, Sandholt BV, Keller SH, et al. 64Cu-DOTATATE PET/MRI for detection of activated macrophages in carotid atherosclerotic plaques: studies in patients undergoing endarterectomy. Arterioscler Thromb Vasc Biol 2015;35(7):1699; with permission.)

Transaxial   Coronal

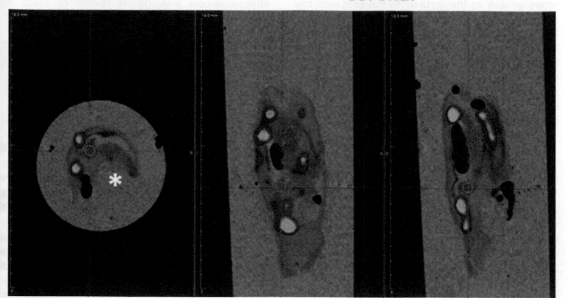

Fig. 3. Ex vivo combined PET/CT visualization of a plaque recovered from the internal carotid artery demonstrating heterogeneous (^{64}Cu) (1,4,7,10-tetraazacyclododecane- *N,N′,N″,N‴*-tetra-acetic acid)-*d*-Phe1,Tyr3-octreotate (^{64}Cu-DOTATATE) uptake 23 hours after injection. Left: transaxial projection of plaque exhibiting hot spots of ^{64}Cu-DOTATATE accumulation. Middle and right: coronal projections at 2 different levels. Residual vessel lumen (*asterisk*). (*From* Pedersen SF, Sandholt BV, Keller SH, et al. ^{64}Cu-DOTATATE PET/MRI for detection of activated macrophages in carotid atherosclerotic plaques: studies in patients undergoing endarterectomy. Arterioscler Thromb Vasc Biol 2015;35(7):1700; with permission.)

expression analyses of selected markers of plaque vulnerability and compared it with ^{64}Cu-DOTATATE uptake, that ^{64}Cu-DOTATATE uptake reflected macrophage load (CD68) but in particular abundance of alternatively activated M2 macrophages (CD163). These macrophages are also known as hemorrhage-associated macrophages and are found in the hemorrhagic part of plaques.[25,26] Because the arterial wall is small compared with the spatial resolution of PET, the use of ^{68}Ga-labeled PET tracers seemed not optimal because of the long positron range (mean range: 3 mm). At least in theory, the much shorter positron range of ^{64}Cu (mean range: <1 mm) would be preferable. Accordingly, the authors compared their newly developed SST$_2$ PET ligand, ^{64}Cu-DOTATATE, which they recently took first in humans,[27,28] in atherosclerosis imaging. They performed a head-to-head comparison with ^{68}Ga-DOTATATOC in 60 patients with cancer without known cardiovascular disease and compared the uptake of both PET tracers in 5 arterial segments with that of the Framingham Risk Score (FRS) of cardiovascular events.[29] Interestingly, the authors found a strong correlation between ^{64}Cu-DOTATATE and FRS (R = 0.4; *P*<.04), whereas no significant

correlation was found between ^{68}Ga-DOTATOC and FRS. These data demonstrate that ^{64}Cu-DOTATATE may be used for risk stratification even in absence of overt plaques, whereas this is not possible with ^{68}Ga-DOTATOC, probably because of differences in radionuclide used. The authors' data indicates that ^{64}Cu-DOTATATE could also become an important tool for monitoring the effect of antiatherosclerotic pharmacologic interventions in the future.

^{18}F-fluorothymidine

From preclinical studies it has been shown that in early stage atherosclerosis, plaque macrophages are recruited from monocytes in the blood.[30] However, in advanced disease macrophages proliferate locally.[30] Accordingly, cell proliferation is expected to be a feature of mature and thereby potentially vulnerable plaques. With the thymidine analogue PET tracer ^{18}F-fluorothymidine (^{18}F-FLT) it is possible to noninvasively demonstrate DNA turnover and thereby cell proliferation. This tracer is used in cancer imaging to provide a noninvasive proliferation index that is sensitive to most types of cancer therapy.[31] Accordingly, the possibility exists that increased ^{18}F-FLT uptake is seen in vulnerable, active plaques. Accordingly, recently the authors compared uptake in both carotid arteries as well as the aorta in 10 patients with low and 10 patients with high FRS.[32] Indeed, they found significantly higher ^{18}F-FLT uptake in the high-risk group. The study compared on a head-to-head basis with that of FDG uptake. As expected, also FDG uptake was higher in the high-risk group; however, there was only a weak correlation between the two PET methods indicating the different information obtained.

[18]F-NaF

The ^{18}F-NaF tracer was originally developed as a PET tracer to be used for bone scintigraphy. ^{18}F-NaF is deposited by chemisorption onto hydroxyapatite and thereby visualizes active calcification. Recently, it has also been applied in imaging of atherosclerotic plaques. Whereas macro-calcification, typically determined by CT, is a measure of plaque burden and does correlate to cardiovascular risk, ^{18}F-NaF PET has the ability to demonstrate the active calcification and mechanism behind the spotty calcifications. The latter may promote plaque vulnerability as it renders the plaque more prone to sheer stress causing microfractures and plaque rupture with subsequent thrombosis.[33] It has been shown that ^{18}F-NaF can identify culprit and ruptured plaques in patients with recent myocardial infarction.[34] ^{18}F-NaF PET correlates with FRS,[33] but there is little overlap with FDG-PET indicating the independent information obtained by the method,[33,35] also with the coronary calcium score there is only a modest correlation with ^{18}F-NaF PET. The latter indicates the importance of discriminating between calcification and active calcification.

Other PET tracers

Based on the pathophysiology of plaque development and instability as well as available PET tracer, the most obvious next-in-line tracers to be tested are angiogenesis and hypoxia tracers. Several new PET tracers for angiogenesis based on the tripeptide RGD are currently being translated into human use. Future studies will show whether the added information will be of any value for risk stratification, treatment selection, and monitoring. Also within hypoxia imaging several tracers are available, for example, ^{18}F-FMISO, ^{18}F-FAZA, and ^{64}Cu-ATSM. For hypoxia tracers, demonstration of added value greater than that of ^{18}F-FDG may be challenging as ^{18}F-FDG is also largely influenced by hypoxia. Accordingly, the authors have shown in oncological settings that little extra information is gained by ^{64}Cu-ATSM if ^{18}F-FDG is also available.[36,37] In addition to the aforementioned, several other tracers have been or are under development for atherosclerosis imaging. A review of these is beyond the scope of this article.

POTENTIAL ADVANTAGES AND CURRENT STATUS OF HYBRID PET/MR IMAGING IN ATHEROSCLEROSIS
An Intriguing Concept and a Perfect Match

Whereas PET and MR each have their key applications and strengths, it is clear that the high cost of a PET/MR imaging scanner, approximately equivalent to that of 3 PET/CT systems, combined with its comparatively low throughput, requires strong arguments for the added value of using PET/MR hybrid imaging for atherosclerosis. However, the methods are surprisingly complementary, building the case for use of hybrid imaging. MR imaging has a high spatial resolution and good tissue contrast necessary for characterization of plaques; PET, on the contrary, only has a modest spatial resolution but a high sensitivity for visualizing molecular targets. Further, PET is a true quantitative method allowing for longitudinal follow-up (eg, when monitoring therapy response). Furthermore, because MR imaging visualizes the vessel wall and plaque rather than the lumen, as is the case with CT, it is possible with higher confidence to delineate on MR imaging the regions of interest where PET data are to be sampled.

Compared with CT, MR imaging is a slow technique particularly if several sequences are used for better tissue characterization. Therefore, MR imaging is best if regional information is to be obtained. This point is exactly what is true for atherosclerotic imaging, whereby typically only the carotid or coronary arteries are to be visualized. In comparison, in most oncological applications whole-body imaging is preferred. Also, the true simultaneous acquisition allows PET and MR imaging to run concomitantly. As hybrid PET/MR systems are relatively new, technical challenges have been many, including the inability to get PET quantification right because no CT-based attenuation map is available.[38–41] However, these problems have now largely been solved; the authors have recently shown in a head-to-head comparison that, for carotid PET, PET/MR and PET/CT quantification is similar.[42] Accordingly, PET/MR imaging for vascular imaging seems ready for prime time.[43] A comparison of strengths of PET/MR and PET/CT for imaging of atherosclerotic plaques is shown in **Table 1**. However, so far very few studies have emerged within this area. Some of these are briefly discussed later.

Table 1
Comparison of strengths of different modalities for imaging of atherosclerotic plaques

	CT	MR	PET	PET/CT	PET/MR
Evaluation of:					
Stenosis	+++	+++	-	+++	+++
Plaque volume	(+)	+++	-	-	+++
Plaque composition (core)	+	+++	-	+	+++
Fibrous cap	-	+++	-	-	+++
Macro-calcification	+++	+	-	+++	+
Microcalcification	-	-	+++	+++	+++
Inflammation (macrophages)	-	+	+++	+++	+++
Angiogenesis	-	(+)	+++	+++	+++
Hypoxia	-	-	+++	+++	+++
Apoptosis	-	-	+++	+++	+++
Feasibility					
Low cost	+++	++	+	++	+
Patient throughput (scan time)	+++	+	++	++	+

+++, Good; ++, Fair; +, Poor; -, N/A.

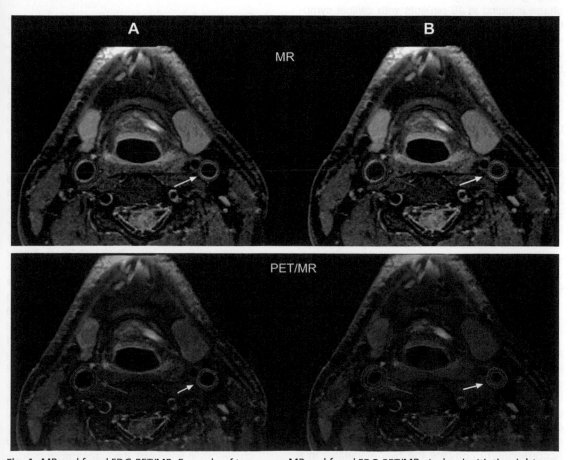

Fig. 4. MR and fused FDG-PET/MR. Example of transverse MR and fused FDG-PET/MR at a level with the right common carotid artery (*red arrow*) and the left internal carotid artery (*white arrow*). A region of interest (ROI) including both the vessel wall and lumen is drawn in column (*A*), and an ROI including only the vessel wall is drawn in column (*B*). (*From* Ripa RS, Knudsen A, Hag AMF, et al. Feasibility of simultaneous PET/MR of the carotid artery: first clinical experience and comparison to PET/CT. Am J Nucl Med Mol Imaging 2013;3(4):364; with permission.)

Hybrid PET/MR Imaging for Vascular Imaging of Atherosclerosis in Humans

Whereas sequential use of PET and MR for imaging of vessels had been described in humans, the authors' group was the first to report the use of simultaneous hybrid PET/MR imaging for arterial wall imaging in humans[42] (**Fig. 4**). The authors studied FDG-PET uptake in the wall of carotid arteries of patients with human immunodeficiency virus with no known cardiovascular disease. We compared on a head-to-head basis with PET/CT and found no difference in FDG quantification. Accordingly, this study demonstrated the feasibility of PET/MR imaging with FDG for evaluation of atherosclerosis. Since then 2 other studies have been published on the quantification of FDG uptake using PET/MR.[44,45] More recently, the authors expanded their studies of PET/MR imaging into the use of non-FDG-PET in a PET/MR imaging study using ^{64}Cu-DOTATATE for macrophage imaging in 10 patients with clinical symptoms of stroke or transient ischemic attack and scheduled for endarterectomy.[24] All patients were ^{64}Cu-DOTATATE-PET/MR imaging scanned before operation, and plaques were recovered for molecular analyses and compared with imaging results. As mentioned earlier, the authors found higher uptake from the symptomatic carotid artery plaque compared with the contralateral side. Also molecular analyses revealed that ^{64}Cu-DOTATATE uptake reflected hemorrhage-associated macrophage load (for details, see earlier discussion). With this study, the authors have opened a field of great potential whereby specific PET tracers are combined with the morphologic and functional information of simultaneously obtained MR. To the best of their knowledge, only 2 other studies using simultaneously acquired PET/MR in imaging of vessel walls have been published since then.[46,47] Both of these studies used FDG as PET tracer.

SUMMARY

Both MR imaging and more recently PET have been established as valuable imaging tools to characterize atherosclerosis and plaque vulnerability. Both within MR and PET work is currently undertaken to develop improved, fast MR sequences and new, specific PET tracers for key markers of atherosclerosis and vulnerability. Accordingly, to combine the two modalities in a one-stop shop using the commercially available hybrid PET/MR imaging scanners seems obvious. Initial technical problems with attenuation correction for PET when using PET/MR hybrid scanners have now largely been solved; in the authors'

view, there are no major obstacles for adaptation of use of hybrid PET/MR imaging in this area. Nevertheless and much to the authors' surprise, they have not yet seen such fast adaptation taking place; only very few studies have been published. It could be that PET/MR was initially anticipated to mainly serve within oncology and neurology and less for vascular evaluation. This view may now be changing, and the authors can only encourage increasing the use of PET/MR for imaging of atherosclerosis and characterization of atherosclerotic plaques.

ACKNOWLEDGMENTS

All of the staff in the PET center is thanked for their skillful assistance.

REFERENCES

1. Chaturvedi S, Bruno A, Feasby T, et al. Carotid endarterectomy–an evidence-based review: report of the therapeutics and Technology assessment Subcommittee of the American Academy of Neurology. Neurology 2005;65(6):794–801.
2. Bailey DL, Pichler BJ, Gückel B, et al. Combined PET/MRI: multi-modality multi-parametric imaging is here: summary report of the 4th International Workshop on PET/MR Imaging; February 23-27, 2015, Tübingen, Germany. Mol Imaging Biol 2015; 17(5):595–608.
3. Dweck MR, Puntman V, Vesey AT, et al. MR imaging of coronary arteries and plaques. JACC Cardiovasc Imaging 2016;9(3):306–16.
4. Kerwin WS, O'Brien KD, Ferguson MS, et al. Inflammation in carotid atherosclerotic plaque: a dynamic contrast-enhanced MR imaging study. Radiology 2006;241(2):459–68.
5. Tang TY, Howarth SPS, Miller SR, et al. The ATHEROMA (Atorvastatin Therapy: Effects on Reduction of Macrophage Activity) Study. Evaluation using ultrasmall superparamagnetic iron oxide-enhanced magnetic resonance imaging in carotid disease. J Am Coll Cardiol 2009;53(22):2039–50.
6. Tang T, Howarth SPS, Miller SR, et al. Assessment of inflammatory burden contralateral to the symptomatic carotid stenosis using high-resolution ultrasmall, superparamagnetic iron oxide-enhanced MRI. Stroke 2006;37(9):2266–70.
7. Libby P, Ridker PM, Hansson GK. Progress and challenges in translating the biology of atherosclerosis. Nature 2011;473(7347):317–25.
8. Pedersen SF, Hag AMF, Klausen TL, et al. Positron emission tomography of the vulnerable atherosclerotic plaque in man–a contemporary review. Clin Physiol Funct Imaging 2014;34(6):413–25.

9. Orbay H, Hong H, Zhang Y, et al. Positron emission tomography imaging of atherosclerosis. Theranostics 2013;3(11):894–902.

10. Yun M, Yeh D, Araujo LI, et al. F-18 FDG uptake in the large arteries: a new observation. Clin Nucl Med 2001;26(4):314–9.

11. Rudd JHF, Warburton EA, Fryer TD, et al. Imaging atherosclerotic plaque inflammation with [18F]-fluorodeoxyglucose positron emission tomography. Circulation 2002;105(23):2708–11.

12. Tawakol A, Migrino RQ, Bashian GG, et al. In vivo 18F-fluorodeoxyglucose positron emission tomography imaging provides a noninvasive measure of carotid plaque inflammation in patients. J Am Coll Cardiol 2006;48(9):1818–24.

13. Graebe M, Pedersen SF, Borgwardt L, et al. Molecular pathology in vulnerable carotid plaques: correlation with [18]-fluorodeoxyglucose positron emission tomography (FDG-PET). Eur J Vasc Endovasc Surg 2009;37(6):714–21.

14. Pedersen SF, Graebe M, Fisker Hag AM, et al. Gene expression and 18FDG uptake in atherosclerotic carotid plaques. Nucl Med Commun 2010;31(5):423–9.

15. Folco EJ, Sheikine Y, Rocha VZ, et al. Hypoxia but not inflammation augments glucose uptake in human macrophages: implications for imaging atherosclerosis with 18fluorine-labeled 2-deoxy-D-glucose positron emission tomography. J Am Coll Cardiol 2011;58(6):603–14.

16. Pedersen SF, Græbe M, Hag AMF, et al. (18)F-FDG imaging of human atherosclerotic carotid plaques reflects gene expression of the key hypoxia marker HIF-1α. Am J Nucl Med Mol Imaging 2013;3(5):384–92.

17. Pedersen SF, Graebe M, Hag AMF, et al. Microvessel density but not neoangiogenesis is associated with 18F-FDG uptake in human atherosclerotic carotid plaques. Mol Imaging Biol 2012;14(3):384–92.

18. Fayad ZA, Mani V, Woodward M, et al. Safety and efficacy of dalcetrapib on atherosclerotic disease using novel non-invasive multimodality imaging (dal-PLAQUE): a randomised clinical trial. Lancet 2011;378(9802):1547–59.

19. Graebe M, Pedersen SF, Højgaard L, et al. 18FDG PET and ultrasound echolucency in carotid artery plaques. JACC Cardiovasc Imaging 2010;3(3):289–95.

20. Graebe M, Borgwardt L, Højgaard L, et al. When to image carotid plaque inflammation with FDG PET/CT. Nucl Med Commun 2010;31(9):773–9.

21. Armani C, Catalani E, Balbarini A, et al. Expression, pharmacology, and functional role of somatostatin receptor subtypes 1 and 2 in human macrophages. J Leukoc Biol 2007;81(3):845–55.

22. Rominger A, Saam T, Vogl E, et al. In vivo imaging of macrophage activity in the coronary arteries using 68Ga-DOTATATE PET/CT: correlation with coronary calcium burden and risk factors. J Nucl Med 2010; 51(2):193–7.

23. Li X, Samnick S, Lapa C, et al. 68Ga-DOTATATE PET/CT for the detection of inflammation of large arteries: correlation with18F-FDG, calcium burden and risk factors. EJNMMI Res 2012;2(1):52.

24. Pedersen SF, Sandholt BV, Keller SH, et al. 64Cu-DOTATATE PET/MRI for detection of activated macrophages in carotid atherosclerotic plaques: studies in patients undergoing endarterectomy. Arterioscler Thromb Vasc Biol 2015;35(7):1696–703.

25. Boyle JJ, Harrington HA, Piper E, et al. Coronary intraplaque hemorrhage evokes a novel atheroprotective macrophage phenotype. Am J Pathol 2009; 174(3):1097–108.

26. Finn AV, Nakano M, Polavarapu R, et al. Hemoglobin directs macrophage differentiation and prevents foam cell formation in human atherosclerotic plaques. J Am Coll Cardiol 2012;59(2):166–77.

27. Pfeifer A, Knigge U, Mortensen J, et al. Clinical PET of neuroendocrine tumors using 64Cu-DOTATATE: first-in-humans study. J Nucl Med 2012;53(8):1207–15.

28. Pfeifer A, Knigge U, Binderup T, et al. 64Cu-DOTATATE PET for neuroendocrine tumors: a prospective head-to-head comparison with 111In-DTPA-Octreotide in 112 patients. J Nucl Med 2015;56(6):847–54.

29. Malmberg C, Ripa RS, Johnbeck CB, et al. 64Cu-DOTATATE for noninvasive assessment of atherosclerosis in large arteries and its correlation with risk factors: head-to-head comparison with 68Ga-DOTATOC in 60 patients. J Nucl Med 2015;56(12):1895–900.

30. Robbins CS, Hilgendorf I, Weber GF, et al. Local proliferation dominates lesional macrophage accumulation in atherosclerosis. Nat Med 2013;19(9):1166–72.

31. Jensen MM, Kjaer A. Monitoring of anti-cancer treatment with (18)F-FDG and (18)F-FLT PET: a comprehensive review of pre-clinical studies. Am J Nucl Med Mol Imaging 2015;5(5):431–56.

32. Ye Y-X, Calcagno C, Binderup T, et al. Imaging macrophage and hematopoietic progenitor proliferation in atherosclerosis. Circ Res 2015;117(10):835–45.

33. Dweck MR, Chow MWL, Joshi NV, et al. Coronary arterial 18F-sodium fluoride uptake: a novel marker of plaque biology. J Am Coll Cardiol 2012;59(17):1539–48.

34. Joshi NV, Vesey AT, Williams MC, et al. 18F-fluoride positron emission tomography for identification of ruptured and high-risk coronary atherosclerotic plaques: a prospective clinical trial. Lancet 2014; 383(9918):705–13.

35. Derlin T, Tóth Z, Papp L, et al. Correlation of inflammation assessed by 18F-FDG PET, active mineral

deposition assessed by 18F-fluoride PET, and vascular calcification in atherosclerotic plaque: a dual-tracer PET/CT study. J Nucl Med 2011;52(7): 1020–7.

36. Hansen AE, Kristensen AT, Jørgensen JT, et al. (64) Cu-ATSM and (18)FDG PET uptake and (64)Cu-ATSM autoradiography in spontaneous canine tumors: comparison with pimonidazole hypoxia immunohistochemistry. Radiat Oncol 2012;7:89.

37. Hansen AE, Kristensen AT, Law I, et al. Multimodality functional imaging of spontaneous canine tumors using 64Cu-ATSM and 18FDG PET/CT and dynamic contrast enhanced perfusion CT. Radiother Oncol 2012;102(3):424–8.

38. Andersen FL, Ladefoged CN, Beyer T, et al. Combined PET/MR imaging in neurology: MR-based attenuation correction implies a strong spatial bias when ignoring bone. Neuroimage 2014;84:206–16.

39. Ladefoged CN, Hansen AE, Keller SH, et al. Dental artifacts in the head and neck region: implications for Dixon-based attenuation correction in PET/MR. EJNMMI Phys 2015;2(1):8.

40. Ladefoged CN, Hansen AE, Keller SH, et al. Impact of incorrect tissue classification in Dixon-based MR-AC: fat-water tissue inversion. EJNMMI Phys 2014; 1(1):101.

41. Ladefoged CN, Benoit D, Law I, et al. Region specific optimization of continuous linear attenuation coefficients based on UTE (RESOLUTE): application to PET/MR brain imaging. Phys Med Biol 2015;60(20) 8047–65.

42. Ripa RS, Knudsen A, Hag AMF, et al. Feasibility o simultaneous PET/MR of the carotid artery: first clinical experience and comparison to PET/CT. Am J Nucl Med Mol Imaging 2013;3(4):361–71.

43. Ripa RS, Kjær A. Imaging atherosclerosis with hybrid positron emission tomography/magnetic resonance imaging. Biomed Res Int 2015;2015 914516.

44. Bini J, Robson PM, Calcagno C, et al. Quantitative carotid PET/MR imaging: clinical evaluation of MR-attenuation correction versus CT-attenuation correction in (18)F-FDG PET/MR emission data and comparison to PET/CT. Am J Nucl Med Mol Imaging 2015;5(3):293–304.

45. Bini J, Eldib M, Robson PM, et al. Simultaneous carotid PET/MR: feasibility and improvement of magnetic resonance-based attenuation correction. Int J Cardiovasc Imaging 2016;32(1):61–71.

46. Li X, Heber D, Rausch I, et al. Quantitative assessment of atherosclerotic plaques on (18)F-FDG PET/ MRI: comparison with a PET/CT hybrid system. Eur J Nucl Med Mol Imaging 2016;43(8):1503–12.

47. Hyafil F, Schindler A, Sepp D, et al. High-risk plaque features can be detected in non-stenotic carotid plaques of patients with ischaemic stroke classified as cryptogenic using combined (18)F-FDG PET/MR imaging. Eur J Nucl Med Mol Imaging 2016;43(2): 270–9.

Clinical PET/MR Imaging in Oncology
Future Perspectives

Andreas Kjær, MD, PhD, DMSc[a],*, Drew A. Torigian, MD, MA, FSAR[b]

KEYWORDS

- PET/MR imaging • Molecular imaging • HyperPET • Cancer

KEY POINTS

- PET/MR imaging will likely not replace PET/computed tomography (CT) as the workhorse for cancer imaging.
- Prostate, breast, brain, and musculoskeletal malignancies are entities whereby PET/MR imaging may play an increasingly important role in clinical practice relative to PET/CT.
- Combined functional MR imaging and molecular PET may be valuable.
- Radiomics using hybrid PET/MR imaging data may support implementation of precision medicine in oncology.
- HyperPET, the combination of hyperpolarized magnetic resonance spectroscopy and PET, may be valuable in cancer phenotyping.

INTRODUCTION

When fully integrated clinical PET/MR imaging systems became available in 2011,[1,2] many radiologists and nuclear medicine physicians thought these scanners would replace PET/computed tomography (CT) systems. Accordingly, an ever-increasing number of PET/MR imaging scanners were expected to be installed. Today, we know this has in no way been the case, as still less than 100 hybrid systems are installed worldwide. The reasons for this are numerous, some of which were first realized when these systems came into routine use. Firstly, the price of PET/MR imaging systems is still substantial, costing more than that of 3 state-of-the-art PET/CT systems. Accordingly, substantial advantages above patient comfort and convenience are necessary to justify the investment. Second, PET/MR imaging is in many ways a regional imaging technique, which limits the types of diseases where it is practical to use. Third, PET/MR imaging is a slow technique with long protocols and low patient throughput. Finally, during the infancy of commercial PET/MR imaging systems, technical issues with attenuation correction, and thereby PET quantification, were problematic.[3,4] However, these have largely been solved by now.

The authors have nothing to disclose.
Dr A. Kjær has received generous support from the John & Birthe Meyer Foundation, the National Advanced Technology Foundation, the Innovation Fund Denmark, the Danish Medical Research Council, the Rigshospitalets Research Foundation, the Svend Andersen Foundation, the AP Møller Foundation, the Novo Nordisk Foundation, and the Lundbeck Foundation to perform the studies reported here.

[a] Department of Clinical Physiology, Nuclear Medicine & PET and Cluster for Molecular Imaging, Rigshospitalet and University of Copenhagen, Denmark; [b] Department of Radiology, Hospital of the University of Pennsylvania, 3400 Spruce Street, Philadelphia, PA 19104, USA
* Corresponding author. Department of Clinical Physiology, Nuclear Medicine & PET, Rigshospitalet, KF-4012, Blegdamsvej 9, Copenhagen 2100, Denmark.
E-mail address: akjaer@sund.ku.dk

PET Clin 11 (2016) 489–493
http://dx.doi.org/10.1016/j.cpet.2016.05.010
1556-8598/16/$ – see front matter © 2016 Elsevier Inc. All rights reserved.

Taken together, it is, therefore, clear that the future of PET/MR imaging lies in applications that give substantial additional and important information above what PET/CT or sequentially performed PET and MR imaging are capable of. The authors discuss areas where PET/MR imaging may be justified and have a bright future, predominantly focusing on oncologic applications. Also, areas where the authors do not think PET/MR imaging will play a role in the future are discussed.

PET/MR IMAGING AS A REPLACEMENT FOR PET/CT IN ROUTINE ASSESSMENT IN ONCOLOGIC CLINICAL PRACTICE

Recently, Spick and colleagues[5] published a review on whether ^{18}F-2-fluoro-2-deoxy-D-glucose (FDG) PET/MR imaging improves cancer assessment compared with FDG PET/CT. In this review, which was based on published studies of more than 2300 patients, in almost any type of cancer there was no advantage of using PET/MR imaging if merely using MR imaging for imaging morphology instead of CT. Accordingly, the authors do not believe in any substantial increase in such use of PET/MR imaging. However, in pediatric oncology, the lower radiation dose burden may justify its use on a routine basis.[6] Furthermore, in some selected cancer types, such as prostate cancer, where MR imaging is increasingly used and much better than CT, PET/MR imaging may be increasingly used.[7–10] This increased use is also driven by the notion that more advanced MR imaging techniques may be valuable in this disease. Please note that prostate cancer represents a clinical entity where regional imaging is valuable and thereby protocol time may be reasonable. For similar reasons, PET/MR imaging may play an increasingly important role in the evaluation of breast, brain, and musculoskeletal malignancies.

WHEN PET/MR IMAGING PROVIDES COMPLEMENTARY INFORMATION

The real advantage and justification of PET/MR imaging lies in combining information from the 2 modalities that are complementary and typically of functional and molecular character. Examples include the use of diffusion-weighted MR imaging (DWI) and dynamic contrast-enhanced MR imaging for assessment of lesion cellularity and perfusion, respectively, in combination with various PET radiotracers. Accordingly, DWI and fluorine-18-fluorothymidine PET for assessment of cellularity may improve phenotyping of cancer lesions.

For prostate cancer, gallium-68-prostate–specific membrane antigen (PSMA) may be an interesting radiotracer to use in the future with PET/MR imaging.[7] In many cases, evaluation of newly developed PET radiotracers may best be performed using PET/MR imaging. As an example, one of the authors recently developed a new PET radiotracer for visualization of the aggressive tumor phenotype based on targeting the urokinase-type plasminogen activator receptor (uPAR).[11] In a phase I study, 3 different cancer types were imaged with PET/CT using a radiotracer targeted toward uPAR.[12] However, in the planned phase II studies, PET/MR imaging will be used to compare uPAR PET with various MR imaging readouts. For PET imaging of angiogenesis, for example, in glioblastomas, PET/MR imaging may also be an obvious choice with use of various MR imaging sequences and readouts for determining perfusion and cell density.

For many years, development of multimodality probes has been ongoing. However, although impressive when applied in preclinical studies, this does not really serve the purpose of obtaining complementary data. Also, when PET and MR imaging are both available, specific PET probes are the preferred choice rather than MR imaging probes, given that PET is much more sensitive than MR imaging and often allows for microdosing.

MULTIPARAMETRIC PET/MR IMAGING AND RADIOMICS

Another field of future clinical potential involves the use of quantitative, parametric imaging both with PET and MR imaging. For MR imaging, several parameters may be obtained. When parametric data from PET and MR imaging are combined, a much-improved phenotyping of cancer is possible that may serve to support the practice of *precision medicine* in oncology. If such data are available on a voxel-to-voxel basis, large data sets may emerge whereby visual qualitative assessment is insufficient to extract all information. Here, data mining of the large data sets is necessary. This exciting field, known as *radiomics*, may hold great promise for optimized tissue characterization and phenotyping.[13,14] The field is still in its infancy, but activities are ongoing to promote this area and to exploit possible advantages. It may be that it proves particularly valuable in radiation therapy planning, where the PET community for many years has suggested *dose-painting by numbers*, a concept, which it is fair to say, that has not been implemented in everyday routine radiation planning.

THE POTENTIAL ROLE OF HyperPET

An interesting concept to take PET/MR imaging to the next level is the possibility of combining hyperpolarized magnetic resonance spectroscopy (MRS) and PET, which has been named hyperPET by one of the authors.[15]

Hyperpolarized MRS is a technique whereby ^{13}C-containing biological compounds are hyperpolarized using a commercially available hyperpolarizer before administration. In this way, the nuclear polarization is increased by about 10,000 fold and the compound can be measured by MRS.[16] The most commonly used compound is ^{13}C-pyruvate whereby the Warburg effect can be followed by the conversion of ^{13}C-pyruvate to ^{13}C-lactate[17] (**Fig. 1**). MRS imaging of the ^{13}C-pyruvate to ^{13}C-lactate conversion was recently used first in humans in patients with prostate cancer.[18]

One of the authors recently demonstrated in companion dogs with spontaneous tumors the feasibility of combining hyperpolarized MRS with FDG PET.[15,19] From these studies, it could clearly

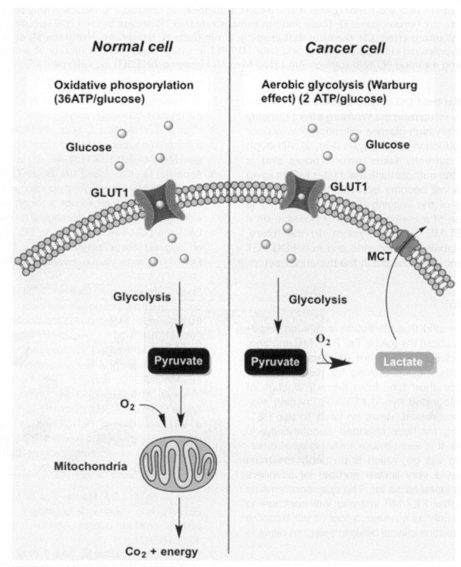

Fig. 1. Warburg effect. In cancer cells, a switch to glycolysis with production of lactate even in the presence of sufficient oxygen (O_2) is seen. This effect is called the Warburg effect. CO_2, carbon dioxide; GLUT1, glucose transporter 1; MCT, monocarboxylate transporter. (*From* Gutte H, Hansen AE, Henriksen ST, et al. Simultaneous hyperpolarized (13)C-pyruvate MRI and (18)F-FDG PET in cancer (hyperPET): feasibility of a new imaging concept using a clinical PET/MRI scanner. Am J Nucl Med Mol Imaging 2015;5(1):39; with permission.)

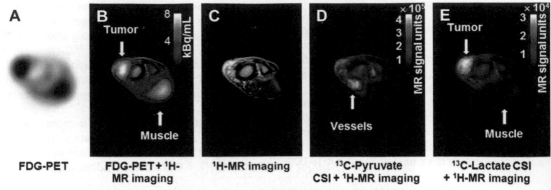

Fig. 2. HyperPET of spontaneous liposarcoma in right front leg of Labrador dog. Note the high concentration of FDG in both muscle and tumor (*panel A* and *arrows* in *panel B*). In contrast, ^{13}C-lactate is only seen in tumor and not in muscle (*arrows, panel E*). These findings demonstrate that ^{13}C-lactate but not FDG specifically demonstrates the Warburg effect. CSI, chemical shift imaging. (*From* Gutte H, Hansen AE, Henriksen ST, et al. Simultaneous hyperpolarized (13)C-pyruvate MRI and (18)F-FDG PET in cancer (hyperPET): feasibility of a new imaging concept using a clinical PET/MRI scanner. Am J Nucl Med Mol Imaging 2015;5(1):42; with permission.)

be seen that the FDG uptake studied by PET was not directly visualizing the Warburg effect but only the secondary high glucose utilization due to poor energy production of glycolysis (**Fig. 2**). Although hyperPET currently takes several hours and is laborious, the authors think that faster MR imaging sequences will become available that will lead to shortening of the imaging protocol. HyperPET is an example of a methodology only possible on a hybrid PET/MR imaging system. In the future, other ^{13}C-labeled compounds and non–FDG PET radiotracers will be tested in the hyperPET setup.

SUMMARY

It has been said that prediction is difficult, especially if it is about the future. For PET/MR imaging, its future clinical role is not obvious, as it is a technique that is still looking for niche applications. In the short time from the introduction of the fully integrated hybrid PET/MR imaging systems to the present, views on what to use PET/MR imaging for have changed substantially. In many ways, it is less obvious today in what direction its use will go, which is probably the main reason that a very limited number of scanners have been installed so far. The question remains as to whether PET/MR imaging will continue to be used mainly as a research tool or will become used on a routine clinical basis in selected disease entities.

REFERENCES

1. Delso G, Fürst S, Jakoby B, et al. Performance measurements of the Siemens mMR integrated whole-body PET/MR scanner. J Nucl Med 2011; 52(12):1914–22.

2. Kjær A, Loft A, Law I, et al. PET/MRI in cancer patients: first experiences and vision from Copenhagen. MAGMA 2013;26(1):37–47.

3. Andersen FL, Ladefoged CN, Beyer T, et al. Combined PET/MR imaging in neurology: MR-based attenuation correction implies a strong spatial bias when ignoring bone. Neuroimage 2014;84:206–16.

4. Ladefoged CN, Hansen AE, Keller SH, et al. Impact of incorrect tissue classification in Dixon-based MR-AC: fat-water tissue inversion. EJNMMI Phys 2014;1(1):101.

5. Spick C, Herrmann K, Czernin J. 18F-FDG PET/CT and PET/MRI perform equally well in cancer: evidence from studies on more than 2,300 patients. J Nucl Med 2016;57(3):420–30.

6. Gatidis S, la Fougère C, Schaefer JF. Pediatric oncologic imaging: a key application of combined PET/MRI. ROFO Fortschr Geb Rontgenstr Nuklearmed 2016;188(4):359–64.

7. Afshar-Oromieh A, Haberkorn U, Schlemmer HP, et al. Comparison of PET/CT and PET/MRI hybrid systems using a 68Ga-labelled PSMA ligand for the diagnosis of recurrent prostate cancer: initial experience. Eur J Nucl Med Mol Imaging 2014; 41(5):887–97.

8. Eiber M, Nekolla SG, Maurer T, et al. (68)Ga-PSMA PET/MR with multimodality image analysis for primary prostate cancer. Abdom Imaging 2015; 40(6):1769–71.

9. Souvatzoglou M, Eiber M, Takei T, et al. Comparison of integrated whole-body [11C] choline PET/MR with PET/CT in patients with prostate cancer. Eur J Nucl Med Mol Imaging 2013;40(10):1486–99.

10. Souvatzoglou M, Eiber M, Martinez-Moeller A, et al. PET/MR in prostate cancer: technical aspects and

potential diagnostic value. Eur J Nucl Med Mol Imaging 2013;40(Suppl 1):S79–88.

11. Persson M, Kjaer A. Urokinase-type plasminogen activator receptor (uPAR) as a promising new imaging target: potential clinical applications. Clin Physiol Funct Imaging 2013;33(5):329–37.

12. Persson M, Skovgaard D, Brandt-Larsen M, et al. First-in-human uPAR PET: imaging of cancer aggressiveness. Theranostics 2015;5(12):1303–16.

13. Kumar V, Gu Y, Basu S, et al. Radiomics: the process and the challenges. Magn Reson Imaging 2012;30(9):1234–48.

14. Lambin P, Rios-Velazquez E, Leijenaar R, et al. Radiomics: extracting more information from medical images using advanced feature analysis. Eur J Cancer (Oxford England 1990) 2012;48(4): 441–6.

15. Gutte H, Hansen AE, Henriksen ST, et al. Simultaneous hyperpolarized (13)C-pyruvate MRI and (18)

F-FDG-PET in cancer (hyperPET): feasibility of a new imaging concept using a clinical PET/MRI scanner. Am J Nucl Med Mol Imaging 2015;5(1):38–45.

16. Ardenkjaer-Larsen JH, Fridlund B, Gram A, et al. Increase in signal-to-noise ratio of >10,000 times in liquid-state NMR. Proc Natl Acad Sci 2003; 100(18):10158–63.

17. Gutte H, Hansen AE, Johannesen HH, et al. The use of dynamic nuclear polarization (13)C-pyruvate MRS in cancer. Am J Nucl Med Mol Imaging 2015;5(5): 548–60.

18. Nelson SJ, Kurhanewicz J, Vigneron DB, et al. Metabolic imaging of patients with prostate cancer using hyperpolarized [1-^{13}C] pyruvate. Sci Transl Med 2013;5(198):198ra108.

19. Gutte H, Hansen AE, Larsen MME, et al. Simultaneous hyperpolarized 13C-pyruvate MRI and 18F-FDG PET (hyperPET) in 10 dogs with cancer. J Nucl Med 2015;56(11):1786–92.

Printed and bound by CPI Group (UK) Ltd, Croydon, CR0 4YY

03/10/2024

01040385-0002